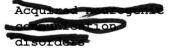
Acquired Neurogenic
Communication Disorders:
A Clinical Perspective

To my parents
Ioannis and Eleni

Acquired Neurogenic Communication Disorders: A Clinical Perspective

Edited by

ILIAS PAPATHANASIOU MSc MRCSLT MCSP

*National Hospital for Neurology & Neurosurgery, London,
and Homerton Hospital NHS Trust, London*

W

WHURR PUBLISHERS

LONDON AND PHILADELPHIA

© 2000 Whurr Publishers
First published 2000 by
Whurr Publishers Ltd
19b Compton Terrace, London N1 2UN, England and
325 Chestnut Street, Philadelphia PA 19106, USA.

British Library Cataloguing in Publication Data
A catalogue record for this book is available from the
British Library.

ISBN: 1 86156 111 3

Printed and bound in the UK by Athenaeum Press Ltd,
Gateshead, Tyne & Wear

Contents

Preface

This book aims to provide an overview of the wide spectrum of approaches that are used to define and describe acquired neurogenic communication disorders, not only from a simple theoretical perspective, but also from a clinical perspective. It is confined to the main aspects of the conditions and does not claim to cover all the dimensions and disciplines contained in the subject. It is based on the collection of presentations by internationally distinguished clinicians at the annual study day of the Specific Interest Group in Adult Neurology (South-East), which took place in September 1998 in London.

The book is divided into two parts. The first section contains four chapters and its focus is on Aphasia and Aphasia Therapy. The first chapter of the section provides an overview of what aphasia is, aphasia therapy and the important issue of efficacy of aphasia therapy. The second chapter gives an overview of the mechanism of recovery of function in aphasia. The third chapter describes the psychosocial framework for therapy intervention in aphasia, issues around the person and how to live with aphasia. In the final chapter of this section, the focus shifts to the cognitive neuropsychological approach to aphasia therapy, analysing in detail the treatment of word retrieval deficits.

In the second section, the topic is Motor Speech Disorders and it also contains four chapters. The first chapter describes the clinical features, the neuroanatomical framework and assessment of dysarthria. The second chapter gives an overview of the model of disablement and how it is used in dysarthria treatment. The third chapter uses a new theoretical framework to describe and define apraxia of speech. Finally, the fourth chapter reviews the instrumentation techniques used in the assessment and therapy of motor speech disorders, with specific focus on case studies using electropalatography.

I hope that this book will provide clinicians, researchers and students with updated clinical and research information on a varied range of topics, covering a wide spectrum of issues.

For the completion of this book, I am grateful to all the contributors from Europe, America and Australia who worked hard to produce the chapters; to the members of the committee of the Specific Interest Group in Adult Neurology (South-East), especially Philippa Clark, Ruth Gilmore, Chris Heron and Helen Ledder, who worked hard to organize the study day; and, finally, many thanks to Renata Whurr for her great support and guidance in the difficult moments of this work.

Ilias Papathanasiou
London 1999

Contributors

David R. Beukelman, Department of Special Education and Communication Disorders, Barkley Memorial Center, University of Nebraska, Lincoln, USA

Sally Byng, Department of Clinical Communication Studies, City University, London, UK

Bill Hardcastle, Department of Speech and Language Sciences, Queen Margaret College, Edinburgh, Scotland

David Howard, Department of Speech, University of Newcastle upon Tyne, Newcastle upon Tyne, UK

Nicholas Miller, Department of Speech, University of Newcastle upon Tyne, Newcastle upon Tyne, UK

Bruce E. Murdoch, Department of Speech Pathology and Audiology, The University of Queensland, Brisbane, Australia

Ilias Papathanasiou, National Hospital for Neurology and Neurosurgery and Institute of Neurology, University College London, and Department of Speech and Language Therapy, Homerton Hospital NHS Trust, London, UK

Susie Parr, Department of Clinical Communication Studies, City University, London, UK

Carole Pound, Department of Clinical Communication Studies, City University, London, UK

Deborah G. Theodoros, Department of Speech Pathology and Audiology, The University of Queensland, Brisbane, Australia

Elizabeth C. Ward, Department of Speech Pathology and Audiology, The University of Queensland, Brisbane, Australia

Robert T. Wertz, Veterans Administration Medical Center and Vanderbilt University School of Medicine, Hearing and Speech Sciences, Nashville, USA

Renata Whurr, National Hospital for Neurology and Neurosurgery and Institute of Neurology, University College London, London, UK

Sara Wood, Department of Speech and Language Sciences, Queen Margaret College, Edinburgh, Scotland

Kathryn M. Yorkston, Department of Rehabilitation Medicine, University of Washington, Seattle, USA

Part I
Aphasia and aphasia therapy

Chapter 1
Aphasia therapy: a clinical framework

ROBERT T. WERTZ

A discussion of aphasia therapy requires cautions, because it may be limited and biased. First, one of the virtues of age is that what you know, you know well, and what you do not know no longer matters. Second, nosology can be confusing, especially the nosology employed in discussing aphasia therapy. Kurt Goldstein (1948) suggested that aphasic people have an impairment of abstract attitude. Aphasiologists have no aversion to the abstract. They use words such as 'framework', 'nature' and 'process' and they never lack attitude. Third, the content that follows may be somewhat parochial; bound by the borders of Boston and San Francisco. American aphasiologists, unfortunately, may be naive in regard to the world literature. This may result from lack of facility in languages, including English. And, fourth, there are probably other cautions that should be listed. These will become obvious in the remarks that follow. So, 'Slow! Erroneous zone ahead!'

The purposes of this chapter are to examine the nature of aphasia, to consider a variety of definitions of aphasia, to list theoretical bases for aphasia therapy, to consider the evidence that supports or rejects the efficacy of treatment for aphasia, and to suggest how changes in service delivery may influence the management of aphasia.

The nature of aphasia

Nature is defined as the intrinsic characteristics and qualities of a person or thing. It is also defined as the aggregate of a person's instincts, penchants and preferences. Here are a few of mine.

Benson and Ardila (1996) tell us that this thing we call aphasia '... is the loss or impairment of language function caused by brain damage' (p.3). Thus, we might infer that the nature of aphasia – its intrinsic characteristics and qualities – comprises a disruption in the use of language as a result of damage to the brain. We might also infer that aphasia is not a loss or impairment of speech and that, without brain

3

damage, there can be no aphasia. Thus, conditions such as apraxia of speech and dysarthria are not aphasia, and the absence of verified brain damage would suggest the absence of aphasia. If only it were that simple.

Confusion about the nature of aphasia results when we explore what we mean by language. If we list the conventional components – phonology, morphology, semantics and syntax – do we require that all or only one or more be impaired to be considered aphasia? Moreover, do we include language disruption in the psychotic thought disorders – schizophrenia and other psychoses? Or, what about the dissolution of language in the dementias? Some (Appell, Kertesz and Fisman, 1982; Au, Albert and Obler, 1988) would call this aphasia. Others (Bayles and Kaszniak, 1987; Rosenbek, LaPointe and Wertz, 1989) would not. And where do we place congenital or developmental language disorders – mental retardation or specific language impairment? Some (Kirshner, 1995) escape this dilemma by requiring aphasia to be '... an acquired disorder of previously intact language ability secondary to brain disease' (p.2).

Even the requirement of brain damage presents problems. For example, do we call the person who presents with a disruption of previously intact language ability but no verifiable brain damage from neurological examination or neuroimaging aphasic? We might, because aphasia could be considered a perceptual phenomenon – apparent to an observer – and not a shade of grey on a CT or MRI scan. Moreover, even in the presence of verified brain damage, what must that damage be – focal, diffuse or focal and diffuse? New ways of looking – computerized axial tomography, magnetic resonance imaging, positron emission tomography, single photon emission computed tomography – do not always resolve the dilemma. The gain in brain is not always in the stain.

I have ignored a word – function – in Benson and Ardila's (1996) definition. The World Health Organization's (WHO) (1980) *International Classification of Impairments, Disabilities and Handicaps* implies that 'function' resides under disability. Thus, must one display a disability – reduction in functional communication – to be aphasic? Most aphasic people do, but what if they do not? Does isolated impaired language or isolated handicap constitute aphasia?

A solution to the problem of stating the nature of aphasia is to say that aphasia is what aphasiologists say it is. Or, we could adopt the United States Supreme Court's position on pornography – 'We don't know how to define it, but we know it when we see it.' However, for the purposes of what follows, let us assume that the nature of aphasia is an acquired disorder of previously intact language ability secondary to brain damage. And, the disorder of language may be present as impairment – disruption in phonology, morphology, semantics and/or syntax; disability – a reduction of functional communication in everyday life; and/or handicap – restricted participation in society that reduces the quality of life. And, to provide flexibility, let us assume that the brain damage believed to cause aphasia may be inferred when not verified and that severity of language impairment, disability and handicap need not be equal in each domain.

There is a need for a position, but that position should not be so rigid that it prevents flexibility. For example, Figure 1.1 represents five potential conditions that may occur in or around what might be called 'the nature of aphasic space'. Condition 1 may be the typical aphasic person. The presence of brain damage is verified, and there is essentially equal language impairment, disrupted functional communication and psychosocial handicap. All reside within the nature of aphasic space. Similarly, condition 2 implies that all components that constitute aphasia – brain damage, impairment, disability and handicap – reside within the nature of aphasic space. However, language impairment is disproportional to disability and handicap. Condition 3 indicates that all components are present except verified brain damage. If we consider aphasia to be a perceived phenomenon and the characteristics of impairment, disability and handicap meet the criteria for aphasia and other disorders – dementia, psychoses, malingering and so on – have been ruled out, condition 3 would be considered aphasic. Condition 4 meets only one criterion – verifiable brain damage. There is no language impairment, disability or handicap. Thus, condition 4 would not be considered aphasia. Finally, condition 5 meets two criteria – verified brain damage and language impairment. There is no indication of disability or handicap. The presence of brain damage and language impairment would qualify the condition as aphasic. Of course, additional configurations in this simplistic conception of the nature of aphasic space are possible, for example, verified brain damage resulting in minimal impairment and disability but inordinate handicap. Each of the profiles in Figure 1.1 represents an aphasic person, or a non-aphasic person (condition 4), I have met during the past 35 years.

If we illustrate the nature of aphasia in this manner, the therapeutic goal is to reduce the volume of impairment, disability and handicap within the nature of aphasic space or, if possible, move one or more of the components outside of aphasic space. Brain damage, when verified, will remain. However, that is not a problem, because aphasia is not a hole in the nervous system. What remains is to describe what constitutes language impairment, disability and handicap and, ultimately, how to reduce or mend them. That is done by one's definition of aphasia and the theory and therapy the definition might dictate. We do not lack those definitions, theories and therapies.

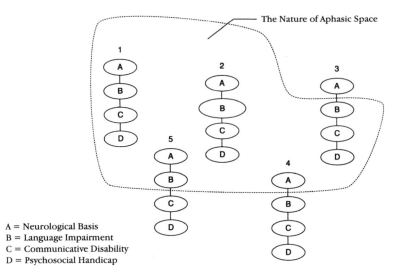

Figure 1.1: The nature of aphasic space showing a variety of characteristics – A=neurological basis, B=language impairment, C=communicative disability, D=psychosocial handicap – as they might exist in a variety of aphasic or non-aphasic people, 1–5.

Aphasia defined

Aphasiologists are always in negotiation with the past, even as they embrace the present and plan the future. Aphasiology's past has provided a variety of definitions of aphasia; new ones emerge frequently; and the future, probably, will perpetuate the practice. Each definition will elaborate the nature of aphasia, identify who we call aphasic, and dictate his or her management. Benson and Ardila's definition (see p. 3) is terse. Others are not so reticent. Four elaborations are considered below.

A general language disorder

Darley (1982) and Schuell and colleagues (1964) eschewed modifying aphasia with adjectives. For Darley, aphasia is:

> Impairment, as a result of brain damage, of the capacity for interpretation and formulation of language symbols; multimodality loss or reduction in efficiency of the ability to decode and encode conventional meaningful linguistic elements (morphemes and larger syntactic units); disproportionate to impairment of other intellective functions; not attributable to dementia, confusion, sensory loss, or motor dysfunction; and manifested in reduced availability of vocabulary, reduced efficiency in application of syntactic rules, reduced auditory retention span, and impaired efficiency in input and output channel selection (p.42).

His definition tells us what he believes aphasia is and what he believes it is not. Differences among aphasic people, for Darley, are represented by differences in severity or the presence of a coexisting disorder, for example, apraxia of speech.

For Schuell et al., aphasia is:

> A general language deficit that crosses all language modalities and may be complicated by other sequela of brain damage (1965: 113).

Thus, Schuell and colleagues' aphasic person would display deficits in auditory comprehension, reading, oral expressive language and writing. Impairment need not be equal in each modality, and depending on severity and time post-onset, an aphasic person may have evolved out of impairments in some modalities.

Aphasia with adjectives

Kertesz (1979), Goodglass and Kaplan (1983), Helm-Estabrooks and Albert (1991) and Damasio (1992), imply that aphasia has a possible selectivity for particular modalities of input and output and, in some instances, for specific input and output combinations. Goodglass and Kaplan (1983) provide a representative definition for this point of view. For them, aphasia is:

> ... the disturbance of any or all of the skills, associations, or habits of spoken or written language, produced by injury to certain brain areas that are specialized for these functions (p.5).

Thus, Goodglass and Kaplan's aphasic person may display deficits in one or more modalities, and the pattern of these deficits permits assigning an adjective – global, Broca's, Wernicke's, Conduction and so on – to describe the pattern observed. Moreover, the pattern often implies the localization of the brain damage that caused the aphasia and the functional interaction of various parts of the nervous system.

Impaired access, resource allocation and attention

Some researchers (Kreindler and Fradis, 1968; McNeil, 1982) provide a definition that emphasizes impaired access to language ability rather than a loss or impairment of language ability. For example, McNeil (1982) said:

> Aphasia is a multimodality physiological inefficiency with, greater than loss of, verbal symbolic manipulations (e.g., association, storage, retrieval, and rule implementation). In isolated form it is caused by focal brain damage to cortical and/or subcortical structures of the hemisphere(s) dominant for such symbolic manipulations. It is affected

by and affects other physiological information processing and cognitive processes to the degree that they support, interact with, or are supported by the symbolic deficits (p.693).

More recently, McNeil (1989) and colleagues (McNeil, Odell and Tseng, 1991) have suggested that linguistic deficits seen in aphasia result from a deficit in resource allocation, specifically the allocation of attention. They imply that aphasia results from impairment in the relationship among attention, arousal and language processing units; shared attention among cognitive domains; equal distribution of attention; efficient allocation of attention; and threshold of activation. Their position attempts to explain not only what aphasia is, but also why it occurs.

A cognitive deficit

The position that aphasia is a cognitive deficit has evolved over at least 20 years. Within this evolution is disagreement about whether aphasia is a cognitive problem or a problem in cognition and language (Davis, 1989). Martin (1981) was an early advocate of aphasia representing a disruption of cognitive processing. Using Neisser's (1966) definition of cognition – all processes by which sensory information is transformed, reduced, elaborated, stored, recovered and used – Martin said aphasia 'is the reduction, because of brain damage, of the efficiency of the action and integration of the cognitive processes that support language' (p.66). Others (Brown, 1977; Chapey, 1986) discuss aphasia as a cognitive and language problem. For example, Chapey says aphasia is 'An acquired impairment in language and the cognitive processes which underlie language caused by organic damage to the brain' (p.7).

Davis (1989) objects to the phrase 'language and cognition'. For him, 'aphasia denotes impaired cognition' (p.726). We might infer that Davis believes that cognition is a supraordinate system, and language is a subordinate subsystem, among, perhaps, several subordinate, cognitive subsystems. And, brain damage that results in aphasia disrupts the cognitive subsystem, language, but may not necessarily disrupt other cognitive subsystems, for example, recognition, understanding, memory, thinking and so on.

Two additional disciplines – psycholinguistics and cognitive neuropsychology – have entered the aphasia arena. Both seem to be aligned, at least in part, with a cognitive position on aphasia. While there are differences between psycholinguistic and cognitive neuropsychological approaches to aphasia, their orientation and definitions of aphasia seem similar. Ratner and Gleason (1993) say that psycholinguistics 'is concerned with discovering the psychological processes that make it possible for humans to acquire and use language' (p.3). Ellis and Young (1988) state that one objective of cognitive neuropsychology is 'to draw conclusions about normal, intact cognitive processes' (p.4). Both employ models of mental processes believed necessary for language. Typically, the models separate components, or modules, into linguistic domains – for example, phonology, semantics and syntax – or language modalities – for example, auditory comprehension, reading, speaking and writing (Lesser, 1987). The rationale, explained by Caramazza and Hillis (1992), is to 'formulate plausible hypotheses about functional lesions to a cognitive system such that the damaged system can explain the observed patterns of impaired performance' and permit taking 'such performance to be consistent with the proposed model of normal cognition' (p.65). Thus, psycholinguistic and cognitive neuropsychological approaches to aphasia seem to define aphasia as a disruption in a psycholinguistic or cognitive neuropsychological model of normal language.

Summary

The above is a sample of definitions of aphasia; not a summary. An apparent omission is a 'functional' or 'pragmatic' definition of aphasia. However, those researchers who advocate a functional or pragmatic approach to treatment, for example, Davis and Wilcox (1981, 1985), do not necessarily define aphasia functionally or pragmatically. For example, Davis (1993) is firmly entrenched in a functional-pragmatic approach to managing aphasia, but he defines aphasia as 'an acquired impairment of the cognitive system for comprehending and formulating language, leaving other cognitive capacities relatively intact' (p.10).

The definitions presented above are certainly more complex than indicated by my abbreviated presentation. Nevertheless, each takes a specific view and elaborates what might be called the nature of aphasia. And, each permits a specific theoretical basis for treating aphasia. Thus, the way one defines aphasia prescribes the nature of aphasia and, usually, how it might be mended. The divergence in definitions implies that aphasiologists' mode of communication is like underwater sonar – each of us bouncing pulses off the other and listening for an echo.

Theoretical bases for aphasia therapy

Read the literature on the theoretical bases for aphasia therapy or observe a variety of treatment sessions and one may conclude that there are as many theories for aphasia therapy as there are aphasiologists treating aphasia. Reviews by Horner and Loverso (1991) and Horner, Loverso and Gonzalez Rothi (1994) on models of aphasia treatment imply that this is a faulty assumption. Some clinicians cluster, with minor differences, in their theoretical approach to treatment, and others treat with no apparent theoretical rationale for their therapy.

What follows is a brief exploration of four theoretical bases, or models, for aphasia therapy. They include a stimulation-facilitation approach, a cognitive-neuropsychological and/or psycholinguistic approach, a functional communication approach, and a neurobehavioural approach. The boundaries are somewhat arbitrary, and the inferences are mine. There is overlap and differences from Horner et al.'s (1994) listing of six theoretical models – stimulation-facilitation, modality, linguistic, processing, minor hemisphere mediation, and functional communication. An obvious omission is the theoretical basis that treatments should be designed to combat deficits represented by specific types of aphasia (Helm-Estabrooks and Albert, 1991). However, I believe that this position and its wonderful acronyms (MIT (Melodic Intonation Therapy), VAT (Visual Action Therapy), VCIU (Voluntary Control of Involuntary Utterances), TWA (Treating Wernicke's Aphasia) and so on) may be absorbed under either a stimulation-facilitation or neurobehavioural umbrella – if not neatly, then perhaps roughly. Similarly, what might be called a psychosocial theoretical position may reside within or, at least, abut a functional communication stance. So, how does it seem to me?

Stimulation-facilitation

Robey (1998) has labelled the stimulation-facilitation theoretical basis the 'Schuell-Wepman-Darley Multimodality (SWDM) treatment' based on the individualized, multimodality stimulation hierarchies developed by Schuell et al. (1964), Wepman (1951) and Darley (1982). As summarized by Duffy (1994), the stimulation-facilitation approach considers aphasia to be a multimodality disruption of language: however, deficits in auditory processing are the primary culprit in aphasic communication, and mending them is the focus of treatment. Thus, treatment tasks employ intensive auditory stimulation with meaningful material in a stimulus–response format. Treatment hierarchies are employed to ensure that the stimulus is adequate (LaPointe, 1978) for the aphasic person's level of severity. The treatment's focus is influenced by the patient's performance on a general measure of language impairment, for example, the Minnesota Test for Differential Diagnosis of Aphasia (Schuell, 1965). While mending or strengthening auditory processes is the underlying principle, treatment may attack deficits in any language modality – auditory comprehension, reading, oral-expressive language or writing. Certainly, the treatment is focused on impairment, but, frequently, an assumption is made that reducing impairment will lessen disability and diminish handicap. Horner et al. (1994) suggest that the use of cueing hierarchies to improve word retrieval (Linebaugh and Lehner, 1977) and extended comprehension training (Marshall and Neuburger, 1984) are examples of the stimulation-facilitation theoretical basis in practice.

Cognitive neuropsychological and/or psycholinguistic

Sometimes called a 'theory for therapy' (Holland, 1992; Wertz, in press), the cognitive neuropsychological and/or psycholinguistic approach seems to view aphasia as a modular or relational processing disruption in a model of normal language. Although there may be differences (Lesser, 1987; Davis, 1996) between a cognitive neuropsychological approach and a psycholinguistic approach, I include them together, because the similarities seem to outnumber the differences.

If a psycholinguistic approach is emphasized, the treatment is designed to restore disrupted language by organizing stimuli to mend the linguistic deficits or impaired module in the psycholinguistic model used to identify the deficit. Similarly, if a cognitive neuropsychological approach is emphasized, the treatment is designed to restore or compensate for language-specific or language-related processing deficits in the model of normal cognition used to identify the deficits. Specific methods to identify deficits include the Psycholinguistic Assessments of Language Processing in Aphasia (PALPA) (Kay, Lesser and Coltheart, 1992) or clinician exploration of specific intact and disrupted modules and their connections in the model used.

Both cognitive neuropsychological and psycholinguistic approaches to aphasia therapy use single-case treatment designs to explore facilitation, reorganization and/or relearning (Howard and Hatfield, 1987). As explained by Edmundson and McIntosh (1995), facilitation is a treatment designed to improve access to intact information when the problem is impaired access. Reorganization treatment attempts to reroute processing through intact components in the model to bypass the processing deficit. And, relearning requires learning lost information or lost rules. Again, the treatment focuses on reducing impairment, but one may assume that reducing impairment may reduce disability and handicap or identify the next treatment targets that, when mended, should ultimately reduce impairment and handicap. An example of the psycholinguistic theoretical basis in practice is Thompson, McReynolds and Vance's (1982) matrix training. And an example of the cognitive neuropsychological theoretical basis in practice is Saffran et al.'s (1992) mapping therapy.

Functional communication

Horner et al. (1994) say that a functional communication theoretical basis posits that communication reflects the application of pragmatic rules, unconstrained by modality, linguistic or neurolinguistic considerations. Aphasia results in ineffective or inefficient language use in natural communication contexts. The rationale for treatment is to facilitate more normal communication by emphasizing pragmatic function over linguistic form and to enhance intermodality flexibility, including establishing strategies for circumventing and/or repairing communication breakdowns. Thus, the focus is on functional communication – communicating in context rather than producing specific linguistic content. Proponents of the functional communication theoretical basis include Holland (1978) and Davis and Wilcox (1981, 1985).

Appraisal of functional communicative ability might employ one of the functional communication measures, for example, *Functional Communication Profile* (Sarno, 1969), *Communicative Abilities in Daily Living* (Holland, 1980), *Communicative Effectiveness Index* (Lomas et al., 1989), or the *Functional Assessment of Communication Skills for Adults* (Frattali et al., 1995). The focus of treatment is on reducing disability – restoring functional communication. Examples of the functional communication approach in practice include Davis and Wilcox's (1985) promoting aphasics' communicative effectiveness (PACE) and Holland's (1991) conversational coaching techniques.

Two additional functional approaches include Kagan and Gailey's (1993) training conversation partners for aphasic adults and Lyon and colleagues' (1997) aphasia partners programme. Although these methods are specifically directed at reducing the handicap associated with aphasia, they seem to have an influence on reducing disability.

Neurobehavioural

Advances in basic neuroscience, specifically brain plasticity and its influence on behaviour subsequent to cortical injury, have led Kolb (1992) to suggest that mechanisms used for plasticity are those used for recovery, and better treatments will result from better understanding and identification of the recovery process. While some treatments for aphasia – Melodic Intonation Therapy (Helm-Estabrooks, Nicholas and Morgan, 1989) and intra- and intersystemic reorganization (Luria, 1970) – flirted with Kolb's suggestion, a basic theoretical position was not advocated until recently (Gonzalez Rothi, 1992; Keefe, 1995; Blomert, 1998; Wertz, in press).

Blomert (1998) suggests that most treatments for aphasia are designed to achieve restoration or substitution, implying that aphasia therapy evokes specific, neurobiological changes in the brain. The traditional belief is that the neurobiological mechanisms associated with language improvement in aphasia are vicariation, redundancy and diaschisis. Vicariation suggests that another brain area, which was not previously involved in a specific function, takes over the function when the area responsible for that function is damaged. Redundancy suggests that undamaged neurones in the general area of damage begin to function and compensate for neurones that have been damaged. Diaschisis suggests that brain damage in one area will inhibit performance in a connected, undamaged area, and relief from this inhibition permits the connected, undamaged area to function normally.

A neurobehavioural theory for aphasia therapy, proposed by Gonzalez Rothi (1992), uses two concepts from the brain plasticity literature – restoration and substitution (Lawrence and Stein, 1978). Treatment techniques appropriate for each concept could be drawn from the theoretical positions described above. For example, restoration – physiological recovery at or around the site of the lesion (redundancy) and the removal of functional influences a lesion might have on other areas of the brain (relief from diaschisis) – would be employed early, for example within the first 3 to 6 months post-onset, when restoration is assumed to occur. Treatment techniques designed to enhance substitution – intra- and/or interhemispheric transfer of function (vicariation) – would be used later, for example after 3 to 6 months post-onset.

Specific restoration techniques would focus on reducing language impairment and might include stimulus-response activities designed to restore auditory comprehension, reading, oral-expressive language, and writing or cognitive neuropsychological or psycholinguistic techniques designed to mend the disruption in the normal model of cognition. Emphasis would be placed on massed practice. Substitution techniques would be designed to reduce impairment and disability. If we seek intra- and interhemispheric reorganization to reduce impairment, Luria's (1970) intrasystemic reorganization and, perhaps, Melodic Intonation Therapy (Helm-Estabrooks et al., 1989) might be appropriate. Similarly, intersystemic reorganization by pairing intact gesture with impaired oral expression (Rosenbek, et al., 1989) would seem appropriate. To reduce disability, intra- and interhemispheric reorganization would be sought through pragmatic methods, for example, promoting aphasics' communicative effectiveness (PACE) (Davis and Wilcox, 1981, 1985), which encourages use of all modalities – speech, gesture, writing, drawing – to achieve communication.

Discussion

A listing of the theoretical bases for aphasia therapy can give a misleading impression of what actually occurs in an aphasic person's management. Typically, the evidence and explanation of therapy based on a specific theoretical position result from an experiment designed to test a hypothesis about theory. However, typical management of aphasic people is eclectic and not confined to testing theory.

Byng (1995) asked the impertinent question, 'What do we do when we say we do therapy?' Impertinent questions are the best kind. Usually, they are important, and, usually, they are useful. Table 1.1 lists Byng's answers to her question. Evident in the list is the implication that therapy is not confined to only one of the WHO dimensions – impairment, disability and handicap. Moreover, therapy is not confined to the confines of a clinical cubicle. And, therapy is not directed only at the aphasic person. How do Byng's suggestions fit within the varied theoretical bases explored above?

Table 1.1: The scope of a speech-language therapist's intervention with someone recovering from aphasia. (After Byng, 1995.)

Delineate the uses of language made by the person with aphasia prior to becoming aphasic

Facilitate accommodation to change in communication skills

Investigate the nature and effects of the language deficit with respect to the whole language system

Attempt to remediate the language deficit

Increase the use of all other potential means of communication to support, facilitate and compensate for the impaired language

Enhance the use of the remaining language

Provide opportunity to use newly acquired and emerging language and communication skills in familiar communicative situations

Attempt to change the communication skills of those around the person with aphasia to accommodate the aphasia

---

First, accounting for the uses of language made by the aphasic patient before becoming aphasic may imply that a normal model of language is not a myth, but individuals may employ a normal model of language differently or with different emphasis. Second, delineating the nature and effects of the language deficit on the whole language system cuts to the core of one's theoretical position. One's delineation of the nature and effects of the language deficit on the whole language system will differ depending on one's theoretical orientation – stimulation-facilitation, cognitive neuropsychological and/or psycholinguistic, functional communication, and so on. Third, attempts to remediate the deficits will depend on one's theory of aphasia therapy and the treatment that theory dictates. Fourth, attempts to increase the use of all other potential means of communication to support, facilitate and compensate for the impaired language may imply that all therapy should include doses of functional communication treatment. Fifth, enhancing the remaining language might send one back to one's theoretical position and the techniques that position dictates. Sixth, providing an opportunity to use newly acquired and emerging language skills not only in a clinical environment, but in more natural communication situations implies, again, that all therapy should involve parts of the functional communication approach. Seventh, facilitate adjustment to the loss of communication skills seems to escape all of the theoretical bases discussed above except, perhaps, Lyon and colleagues' (1997) aphasia partners programme. And, similarly, eighth, attempting to change the communication skills of those around the aphasic patient to accommodate the aphasia does not find a home in any theoretical position except that suburb of the functional communication approach inhabited by Kagan and Gailey's (1993) training conversational partners for aphasic people and Lyon and colleagues' (1997) aphasia partners programme.

Thus, restricting a discussion of therapy to only theoretical bases and the methods these dictate may be misleading, because, again, a theory of or for therapy probably constitutes only a fraction of what clinicians do when they say they do therapy. Our world of niches – theories and therapies – aimed at a particular deficit, type of aphasic person, time post-onset, and, perhaps, postal code may have little to do with therapeutic reality or, at least, only a portion of it. When we do therapy, we might ask whether our therapeutic theories are in the making or the marring.

Aphasia therapy: its efficacy

Aphasiologists are interested in whether what they do for aphasic people does any good. Discussions about the worth of aphasia therapy usually involve a recitation of the data provided by treatment studies, arguing the merits of group and single-case designs, quibbling over the nosology, and a lot of Angst. Certainly, reviews on the efficacy of aphasia therapy exist (for example, Darley, 1972; Enderby and Emerson, 1995; Wertz, 1995). And, certainly, opinions differ regarding the answer to the efficacy question. So, what might be added here that might be useful? Perhaps we may want to consider some things about efficacy, in general, that we never knew or knew and forgot – specifically, the phases in outcomes research and the levels of evidence applied to treatment studies.

Five-phase model of outcomes research

Robey and Schultz (1998) observe:

> While there is strong evidence that the treatments of speech-language pathologists and audiologists have generally proved potent as they have been tested, the accepted standards for clinical-outcome testing used throughout the research community (e.g., by other clinical disciplines, regulatory agencies of the federal government, and third party payers) have been mostly ignored (p.787).

Specifically, tests of the efficacy of treatment for aphasia have ignored the traditional five-phase healthcare model of clinical outcome research shown in Table 1.2. The advantages of the model are the demonstration of how a treatment is developed and its efficacy and effectiveness are tested and how the terms efficacy and effectiveness are defined. Robey and Schultz (1998) have explained the objectives and methods in each phase of the model.

Table 1.2: A five-phase healthcare model of clinical outcome research. (After Robey and Schultz, 1998.)

Phase	Objectives
I	Develop critical research hypotheses for testing in Phase III, establish the safety of the treatment, detect the activity of the treatment, determine the minimal dose for evoking activity
II	Formulate and standardize prescription protocols and clinical methods, validate outcome measures, assess the ranges of factors affecting activity, optimize dosage
III	Test the efficacy of the treatment under optimal conditions in a randomized controlled clinical trial
IV	Test the effectiveness of the treatment under typical circumstances; contrast therapeutic effects attributable to different forms of service delivery, levels of clinician training, variations in the population definition
V	Continue effectiveness testing in the context of associated costs; explore cost-effectiveness, consumer satisfaction and quality of life benefits

The objectives in Phase I are to develop the research hypotheses, establish the safety of the treatment and detect the activity of the treatment. All components of the experiment are addressed: What behaviours are to be changed? Does the change have a positive influence on the lives of patients? For whom is the treatment intended? What competencies must clinicians possess? How is the outcome to be indexed? What magnitude of change constitutes a successful outcome? Under what circumstances is the treatment best delivered? What is the safety of the treatment? and What is the minimal dosage? Means for accomplishing Phase I objectives are case studies, single-subject experiments and small group experiments.

If the outcome of Phase I research warrants testing the efficacy of a treatment, the necessary scientific preparations are undertaken in Phase II. Treatment protocols are developed and standardized, outcome measures are developed and validated, the range of factors that may affect the treatment's activity is assessed, and the dosage is optimized. In Phase I, activity of the treatment is detected. In Phase II, activity of the treatment is established – how much of what for whom. Again, case studies, single-subject experiments and small group experiments are appropriate for Phase II.

Phase III research tests the efficacy of the treatment under ideal conditions. It requires large samples and external controls. Phase III requires a priori statistical power analysis to determine sample size. And, because sample size must be large, Phase III research is frequently a multi-centre, clinical trial. The method for Phase III research is the classical, clinical trial that assigns study patients randomly to treatment and no-treatment groups.

Assuming that efficacy is established in Phase III, Phase IV research includes follow-up tests with specified subpopulations and constitutes the initial efforts in testing the treatment's effectiveness – the change to be expected with typical applications to typical patients under typical conditions. Again, large samples from the target population are required; however, control samples are not used in effectiveness research.

After the treatment is introduced to the practising community in Phase IV, Phase V research emphasizes the continuation of effectiveness research. The functional outcome of the treatment is explored – for example, the discharge location of the patients treated, their quality of life, their survival rates. Also, cost-effectiveness is explored to determine the financial value of the treatment, as well as the general value of the treatment – the quality control necessary, consumer satisfaction, quality of life and the value to society.

Again, a virtue of the five-phase model is that it clarifies the nosology used in outcome research. For example, while all phases of the model explore outcome, if we define outcome as a natural result, a consequence or the difference between points in time – for example, a difference in performance between pre- and post-treatment – we discover that outcome is not efficacy, effectiveness or efficiency. Administering an efficacious treatment may influence outcome, but outcome is not efficacy.

The Office of Technology Assessment (1978) says that efficacy is, 'The probability of benefit to individuals in a defined population from a medical technology applied for a given medical problem under ideal conditions of use' (p.16). Three constraints are implied in the definition. First, the statistical inference made in efficacy research applies to a specific population and not a specific individual. Second, a clearly focused treatment protocol is administered to a clearly defined population. And, third, efficacy research requires optimally selected and trained clinicians, optimally selected patients, optimally delivered treatment, optimally structured conditions, optimal measures of change and so on. Thus, an efficacy experiment indicates the possible benefits of the treatment, not the actual benefits.

The Office of Technology Assessment (1978) says that effectiveness is, 'The probability of benefit to individuals in a defined population from a medical technology applied for a given medical problem under average conditions of use' (p.16). Thus, effectiveness research examines clinical outcomes obtained by ordinary clinicians from ordinary patients under the ordinary circumstances of clinical practice. Therefore, effectiveness experiments should be conducted only after the efficacy of a treatment has been established.

Efficiency means acting or producing effectively with a minimum of waste, expense and unnecessary effort. Thus, for two treatments that have been demonstrated to be efficacious and effective, we might compare them to determine which is most efficient, for example, which results in the most improvement with the least expense and effort.

Levels of evidence

More and more consumers of treatment – individuals, government agencies, third-party payers – are requesting a level of evidence to support the benefit of a proposed treatment. Several levels of evidence scales exist. One, developed by the American Academy of Neurology (1994), is shown in Table 1.3. Class I evidence, in this scale, is evidence from one or more well-designed, randomized controlled clinical trials. Class II evidence comes from one or more randomized clinical studies such as case-control, cohort studies and so on. Class III is evidence from expert opinion, non-randomized historical controls, or one or more case reports. Another levels of evidence scale (Birch and Davis and Associates, 1997) indicates that the highest level of evidence comes from a meta-analysis that includes two or more randomized controlled trials and other studies that have good internal and external validity.

Because of single-subject designs' popularity, and confusion regarding their contribution to demonstrating efficacy, we may want to ponder 'whither single-subject designs?' Robey and Schultz (1998) assert:

> ... efficacy is a property of a treatment delivered to a population and infer-ence to a population requires a group experiment. Efficacy does not manifest in an individual and, as single-subject experiments do not provide inference to a population, they do not and cannot index efficacy (p.805).

Placed within a levels of evidence scale, single-subject experiments would provide a third level of evidence in the Birch and Davis scale and Class II or Class III evidence in the American Academy of Neurology scale.

Table 1.3: A level of evidence scale. (After American Academy of Neurology, 1994.)

Level	Evidence
I	One or more well-designed, randomized controlled clinical trials
II	One or more randomized clinical studies such as case control or cohort studies
III	Expert opinion, non-randomized historical controls, or case reports

Efficacy of aphasia treatment

About 60 reports, not including single-subject experiments, on the efficacy, effectiveness or general outcome of aphasia treatment exist. A review of these reports indicates that the treatments tested were not developed systematically through each phase in the five-phase outcomes research model, and none seemed concerned with the level of evidence the design and results supported. However, a level of evidence could be applied to each. More importantly, consensus regarding the value of aphasia treatment and methods to demonstrate that value is lacking.

Three meta-analyses (Whurr, Lorch and Nye, 1992, 1997 and Robey, 1994, 1998) of clinical outcomes in the treatment of aphasia have been reported. A meta-analysis is a mathematical means for synthesizing independent research findings scattered throughout a body of literature. The product is the average effect size and its confidence interval. These permit estimating the degree to which a particular null hypothesis – for example, treatment for aphasia is not effective – is false on the basis of all available evidence. The results of Whurr et al.'s (1992) meta-analysis prompted them to conclude, 'the verdict on efficacy of treatment must remain open' (p.15). Later (Whurr et al., 1997), however, the authors observed, 'This review found that, overall, speech and language therapy for adult aphasics yielded positive results' (p.9). The results of Robey's meta-analyses led him to conclude, 'The results of this meta-analysis are consistent with those of Robey (1994). The accumulated scientific evidence warrants the assertion that, on average, treatment for aphasic persons is effective' (Robey, 1998: 181).

Only two explorations of the efficacy of aphasia therapy, to my knowledge, have used random assignment of study patients to treatment and no-treatment groups, and the results regarding the efficacy of treatment for aphasia differ. Lincoln et al. (1984) observed no significant differences between treatment and no-treatment groups. Conversely, the second VA Cooperative Study (Wertz et al., 1986) found that aphasic patients treated by speech pathologists made significantly more improvement than aphasic patients who were not treated. Several differences between the two studies may explain the difference in results. Lincoln et al.'s study patients included individuals with single and multiple strokes. Two hours of treatment each week for 24 weeks was prescribed. Less than 30% of the treatment group received the amount of treatment prescribed. VA Cooperative Study participants had suffered a single, first, left-hemisphere stroke. Eight to 10 hours of treatment each week for 12 weeks was prescribed. All study patients, included in the compliers-only analysis, received the treatment prescribed. Thus, the Lincoln et al. investigation combined parts of a Phase III investigation – random assignment to treatment and no-treatment groups – and parts of a Phase IV investigation – treatment under ordinary conditions of typical practice. The VA Cooperative Study was a Phase III investigation –

treatment under ideal conditions. One might conclude that the VA Cooperative Study was designed to determine whether treatment can work, and Lincoln et al. investigated whether treatment does work.

Robey and Schultz (1998) argue that single-subject experiments will not demonstrate efficacy. Conversely, Howard (1986) argued that randomized controlled trials are not a suitable method for assessing treatment efficacy and advocated employing single-subject designs. Whurr et al. (1992) list comparison of treatments designs (for example, Meikle et al. 1979; David, Enderby and Bainton, 1982) as evidence that treatment for aphasia is not efficacious. Others (Wertz, 1995) believe that a comparison of treatments design will not demonstrate efficacy or the lack of it, because the absence of a no-treatment group in a comparison of two treatments with unknown efficacy will only indicate whether one treatment is the same as, better than, or worse than the other.

So, what is one to conclude? Not much beyond the obvious observation that aphasiologists cannot get their act together regarding what constitutes evidence to demonstrate efficacy and what is the most appropriate method for collecting that evidence. If a discipline, for example, aphasiology, elects to stray from the traditional, five-phase outcomes research model, it may need to define how it employs the nosology – outcome, efficacy, effectiveness, efficiency; specify the accepted methodology for collecting evidence to demonstrate what the nosology is defined to indicate; and state the levels of evidence required to support the efficacy of its efforts. However, the discipline may want to consider that if its definitions, methodology and levels of evidence differ from those used in the general scientific community, the discipline's pronouncements regarding the efficacy of its efforts will not be accepted and the discipline will look a little silly.

Changes in service delivery

Frattali (1998) paints a less than rosy picture of aphasia treatment's present and future in the United States:

> Health care is being redefined and restructured aggressively to control its spiraling costs. Byproducts of the change include staff reductions, treatment limits, and lower cost alternatives to traditional care. These and other cost-cutting measures will only become more common as various managed care models proliferate and as federally mandated projects develop prospective payment methodologies for medical rehabilitation. Soon, traditional models of clinical practice may become obsolete (pp.241–2).

This has prompted some aphasiologists to fear that they will become extinct before they have been discovered. Below, I list potential limitations on the delivery of treatment to aphasic people, current requirements imposed on the delivery of services, and potential means for coping with change in service delivery. All relate to the management of aphasic people in the United States.

Limitations

The advent of managed care in the United States may impose restrictions that limit services to: 60 days; 10 sessions for speech-language pathology services; 10 sessions for physical therapy, occupational therapy and speech-language pathology services combined; 2 weeks of speech-language pathology services with possible authorization for continued treatment; or treatment dictated by the managed care organization's critical pathway (Frattali, 1998). In the United States, legislation has been passed that places a cap on payment for speech-language pathology *and* physical therapy outpatient services. Aphasic people with coexisting hemiplegia may need to decide if they want to walk or talk.

Requirements

Medicare Intermediary Manual Guidelines (1991) require a speech-language pathologist to write functional goals that reflect the level of communicative independence a patient is expected to achieve outside the therapeutic environment. These goals must reflect the final level the patient is expected to achieve, must be realistic, and must have a positive effect on the quality of the patient's everyday functions. Treatment for aphasia must indicate: an expectation of significant, practical improvement; functional goals to be achieved; the estimated duration and frequency of treatment; patient and family input to the treatment plan; the pre- and post-treatment measures used to document change; and documentation of progress in relationship to the functional goals.

Coping

Essentially, aphasiologists in the United States will be required to do more with less. Unfortunately, what we know about doing aphasia therapy and the results that therapy might achieve provide few resources in coping with change. For example, the outcome data on aphasia treatment indicate that a minimum of three sessions a week for 5 to 6 months (Basso, Capitani and Vignolo, 1979) or eight to 10 sessions a week for 12 weeks (Wertz et al., 1986) is necessary to demonstrate significantly more improvement in treated patients than untreated patients. Conversely, 2 hours a week for 24 weeks or less (Lincoln et al., 1984) results in no significant difference in improvement between treated and untreated patients. Moreover, the results of treatment must attain a 'functional' improvement in communication. The outcome data on aphasia treatment that imply a positive influence of treatment are indexed by improvement on impairment measures. To my knowledge, there is no documented evidence that implies that aphasia treatment results in significantly more improvement in functional communication than no treatment.

So, how do we cope? The research may need to shift towards the practical – documenting functional outcome, exploring dosage – rather than continuing the interesting – exploring theoretical bases for aphasia therapy. Certainly, there is the necessity of documenting change as 'functional' outcome rather than reduced impairment. And if documenting a change in quality of life is required, there is a need to develop quality of life outcome measures that are specific to and appropriate for aphasic people. Finally, it may be essential to explore alternative methods of service delivery, for example, using aphasiologists as consultants to patient and family rather than as the primary treatment provider. Essentially, if the number of bullets in our arsenal is limited, what are the appropriate targets, when do we fire them, and is it more effective to fire them when targets appear rather than early post-onset in a burst? The nature of the question – how much, of what, for whom, when – has changed. The 'how much' is being dictated. Determining the 'what' and 'for whom' may remain within our grasp, and, perhaps, we may be able to negotiate the 'when'. Most of all, we no longer have the luxury of unlimited debate. Perhaps, we have been poor stewards of our previous resources.

Now that aphasia treatment is being driven more by the marketplace than by science, and the 'E' word has become economics rather than efficacy, what do we do? Certainly, science needs to prevail and it is our responsibility to ensure it does. Within the confines of today's service delivery climate, we may want to do what we have avoided in the past; focus on Phases I and II in the outcomes research model. There, we are required to develop the research hypotheses, establish the safety of the treatment, and detect the activity of the treatment. The goal to be attained is dictated – improve functional communication. However, will improvement, assuming that we can demonstrate it under the confines of limited patient contact, have a positive influence on the lives of patients? Collecting outcome data, pre- and post-treatment, is essential. For whom is the treatment intended? A limited number of treatment sessions may benefit some but not others. Perhaps the latter should not be subjected to a treatment that has no benefit. What should the treatment be? Within the confines of limited access, we need to determine which theoretical basis for treatment results in the most functional gain and improvement in the patient's quality of life. The means for answering the questions are the same – case studies, single-subject experiments and small-group experiments.

Aphasiologists must provide the data to answer the essential questions. If they do not, they will be forced to live with answers others make up. If the above seems to come dangerously close to moralizing, you have missed my point. It is moralizing.

Summary

The preceding has been an attempt to define the nature of aphasia, consider definitions of aphasia that elaborate its nature, compare different theoretical bases for aphasia therapy, sift the evidence that demonstrates whether treatment of aphasia does or does not do any good, and ponder how changes in service delivery may change what aphasiologists do. The wonderful discussion provided by a recent clinical forum in *Aphasiology* on diversity in aphasiology (Petheram and Parr, 1998) summarizes differences in how we view the nature of aphasia, how it should be defined and how it should be treated. Given the opportunity, we may not want to over-manage our destiny. Unfortunately, changes in service delivery may be doing that for us. And, if 'confusion about the conceptual basis of aphasia therapy and the resulting tendency to adhere to dominant paradigms must have the effect of diminishing the service which can be offered to aphasic people, and weakening any claim on resources made by those seeking to assist them' (Petheram and Parr, 1998; 445) is correct, aphasiologists may want to wear two hats, one for the marketplace and one for the science. A united position may cope best with crisis. Conversely, diversity may ensure increasing competence.

Aphasiologists have come to recognize in the pages of their literature a civilization, their civilization, in conversation with itself. It is a series of communiqués of a work always in progress. Perhaps that is exactly as it should be.

References

American Academy of Neurology (1994). Assessment: melodic intonation therapy. Neurology 44: 566–8.

Appell J, Kertesz A, Fisman M (1982). A study of language functioning in Alzheimer patients. Brain and Language 17: 73–91.

Au R, Albert ML, Obler LK (1988). The relation of aphasia to dementia. Aphasiology 2: 161–73.

Basso A, Capitani E, Vignolo L (1979). Influence of rehabilitation of language skills in aphasic patients: a controlled study. Archives of Neurology 36: 190–6.

Bayles KA, Kaszniak AW (1987). Communication and Cognition in Normal Aging and Dementia. Boston, MA: Little, Brown.

Benson DF, Ardila A (1996). Aphasia: A Clinical Perspective. New York: Oxford University Press.

Birch and Davis Associates (1997). The State-of-the-Science in Medical Rehabilitation, Volume 1. Falls Church, VA: Birch and Davis Associates.

Blomert L (1998). Recovery from language disorders: interactions between brain and rehabilitation. In Stemmer B, Whitaker H (eds) Handbook of Neurolinguistics. San Diego, CA: Academic Press, pp.547–57.

Brown JW (1977). Mind, Brain and Consciousness: The Neuropsychology of Cognition. New York: Academic Press.

Byng S (1995). What is aphasia therapy? In Code C, Muller D (eds) The Treatment of Aphasia: From Theory to Practice. London: Whurr, pp.3–17.

Caramazza A, Hillis AE (1992). For a theory of remediation of cognitive deficits. National Institute on Deafness and Other Communication Disorders Monograph 2: 65–75.

Chapey R (1986). An introduction to language intervention strategies in adult aphasia. In Chapey R (ed.) Language Intervention Strategies in Adult Aphasia (2nd Edition). Baltimore, MD: Williams & Wilkins, pp.2–11.

Damasio AR (1992). Aphasia. New England Journal of Medicine 326: 531–9.

Darley FL (1972). The efficacy of language rehabilitation in aphasia. Journal of Speech and Hearing Disorders 37: 3–21.

Darley FL (1982). Aphasia. Philadelphia, PA: WB Saunders.

David RM, Enderby P, Bainton D (1982). Treatment of acquired aphasia: speech therapists and volunteers compared. Journal of Neurology, Neurosurgery, and Psychiatry 45: 957–61.

Davis GA (1989). The clinical cloud and language disorders. Aphasiology 3: 723–33.

Davis GA (1993). A Survey of Adult Aphasia and Related Language Disorders (2nd Edition). Englewood Cliffs, NJ: Prentice Hall.

Davis GA (1996). Obligations and options in the evaluation of aphasia. American Speech-Language Hearing Association Division 2, Neurophysiology and Neurogenic Speech and Language Disorders 6: 2–8.

Davis GA, Wilcox J (1981). Incorporating parameters of natural conversation in aphasia. In Chapey R (ed.) Language Intervention Strategies in Adult Aphasia. Baltimore, MD: Williams & Wilkins, pp.169–94.

Davis GA, Wilcox MJ (1985). Adult Aphasia Rehabilitation: Applied Pragmatics. San Diego, CA: College-Hill Press.

Duffy JR (1994). Schuell's stimulation approach to rehabilitation. In Chapey R (ed.) Language Intervention Strategies in Adult Aphasia (3rd Edition). Baltimore, MD: Williams & Wilkins, pp.146–74.

Edmundson A, McIntosh J (1995). Cognitive neuropsychology and aphasia therapy: putting the theory into practice. In Code C, Muller D (eds) The Treatment of Aphasia: From Theory to Practice. London: Whurr, pp.137–63.

Ellis AW, Young AW (1988). Human Cognitive Neuropsychology. Hove: Lawrence Erlbaum.

Enderby P, Emerson J (1995). Does Speech and Language Therapy Work? London: Whurr.

Frattali CM (1998). Clinical care in a changing health system. In Helm-Estabrooks N, Holland AL (eds) Approaches to the Treatment of Aphasia. San Diego, CA: Singular Publishing, pp.241–65.

Frattali CM, Thompson CK, Holland AL, Wohl CB, Ferketic MM (1995). Functional Assessment of Communication Skills for Adults. Rockville, MD: American Speech-Language-Hearing Association.

Goldstein K (1948). Language and Language Disturbances. New York: Grune & Stratton.

Gonzalez Rothi LJ (1992). Theory and clinical intervention: One clinician's view. National Institute on Deafness and Other Communication Disorders Monograph 2: 91–8.

Goodglass H, Kaplan E (1983). The Assessment of Aphasia and Related Disorders (2nd Edition). Philadelphia, PA: Lea & Febiger.

Helm-Estabrooks N, Albert ML (1991). Manual of Aphasia Therapy. Austin, TX: pro-ed.

Helm-Estabrooks N, Nicholas M, Morgan A (1989) Melodic Intonation Therapy Program. San Antonio, TX: Special Press.

Holland AL (1978). Functional communication in the treatment of aphasia. Communicative Disorders: An Audio Journal for Continuing Education 3. New York: Grune & Stratton.

Holland AL (1980). Communicative Abilities in Daily Living. Baltimore, MD: University Park Press.

Holland AL (1991). Pragmatic aspects of intervention in aphasia. Journal of Neurolinguistics 6: 197–211.

Holland AL (1992). Some thoughts on future needs and directions for research and treatment of aphasia. National Institute on Deafness and Other Communication Disorders Monograph 2: 147–52.

Horner J, Loverso FL (1991). Models of aphasia treatment in Clinical Aphasiology 1972–1988. In Prescott TE (ed.) Clinical Aphasiology, Volume 20. Austin, TX: pro-ed, pp.61–75.

Horner J, Loverso FL, Gonzalez Rothi L (1994). Models of aphasia treatment. In Chapey R (ed.) Language Intervention Strategies in Adult Aphasia. Baltimore, MD: Williams & Wilkins, pp.135–45.

Howard D (1986). Beyond randomized controlled trials: the case for effective case studies of the effects of treatment in aphasia. British Journal of Disorders of Communication 21: 89–102.

Howard D, Hatfield FM (1987). Aphasia Therapy: Historical and Contemporary Issues. London: Lawrence Erlbaum.

Kagan A, Gailey GF (1993). Functional is not enough: training conversation partners for aphasic adults. In Holland AL, Forbes MM (eds) Aphasia Treatment: World Perspectives. San Diego, CA: Singular Publishing Group, pp.199–225.

Kay J, Lesser R, Coltheart M (1992). Psycholinguistic Assessments of Language Processing in Aphasia (PALPA). Hove: Lawrence Erlbaum.

Keefe KA (1995). Applying basic neuroscience to aphasia therapy: what the animals are telling us. American Journal of Speech-Language Pathology 4: 88–93.

Kertesz A (1979). Aphasia and Associated Disorders: Taxonomy, Localization, and Recovery. New York: Grune & Stratton.

Kirshner H (1995). Introduction to aphasia. In Kirshner HS (ed.) Handbook of Neurological Speech and Language Disorders. New York: Marcel Dekker, pp.1–21.

Kolb B (1992). Mechanisms underlying recovery from cortical injury: reflections on progress and directions for the future. In Rose FD, Johnson DA (eds) Recovery from Brain Damage. New York: Plenum Press, pp.169–86.

Kreindler A, Fradis A (1968). Performances in Aphasia. A Neurodynamical, Diagnostic and Psychological study. Paris: Gauthier-Villars.

LaPointe LL (1978). Aphasia therapy: some principles and strategies for treatment. In Johns DF (ed.) Clinical Management of Neurogenic Communicative Disorders. Boston, MA: Little, Brown, pp.129–90.

Lawrence S, Stein D (1978). Recovery after brain damage and the concept of localization of function. In Finger S (ed.) Recovery from Brain Damage: Research and Theory. New York: Plenum Press, pp.369–407.

Lesser R (1987). Cognitive neuropsychological influences on aphasia therapy. Aphasiology 1: 189–200.

Lincoln NB, McGuirk E, Mulley GP, Lendrem W, Jones AC, Mitchell JRA (1984). Effectiveness of speech therapy for aphasic stroke patients: a randomized controlled trial. Lancet 1: 1197–200.

Linebaugh CW, Lehner LH (1977). Cuing hierarchies and word retrieval: a therapy program. In Brookshire RH (ed.) Proceedings of the Conference on Clinical Aphasiology. Minneapolis, MN: BRK Publishers, pp.19–31.

Lomas J, Pickard L, Bester S, Finlayson A, Zoghaib C (1989). The communicative effectiveness index: development and psychometric evaluation of a functional communication measure for adult aphasia. Journal of Speech and Hearing Disorders 54: 113–24.

Luria AR (1970). Traumatic Aphasia: Its Syndromes, Psychology, and Treatment. The Hague: Mouton.

Lyon JG, Cariski D, Keisler L, Rosenbek J, Levine R, Kumpula J, Ryff C, Coyne S, Blanc M (1997). Communication partners: enhancing participation in life and communication for adults with aphasia in natural settings. Aphasiology 11: 693–708.

Marshall RC, Neuburger S (1984). Extended comprehension training reconsidered. In Brookshire RH (ed.) Proceedings of the Conference on Clinical Aphasiology. Minneapolis, MN: BRK Publishers, pp.181–7.

Martin AD (1981). The role of theory in therapy: a rationale. Topics in Language Disorders 1: 63–72.

McNeil MR (1982). The nature of aphasia in adults. In Lass NJ, McReynolds LV, Northern JL, Yoder DE (eds) Speech, Language, and Hearing, Volume III. Pathologies of Speech and Language. Philadelphia, PA: WB Saunders, pp.692–740.

McNeil MR (1989) Some theoretical and clinical implications of operating from a formal definition of aphasia. Paper presented to the Academy of Aphasia, Santa Fe, NM.

McNeil MR, Odell K, Tseng CH (1991). Toward the integration of resource allocation into a general theory of aphasia. In Prescott TE (ed.) Clinical Aphasiology, Volume 20. Austin, TX: pro-ed, pp.21–39.

Medicare Intermediary Manual (1991). Part 3 – Claims Process, section 3905, Medical review Part B, intermediary outpatient speech-language pathology bills. Health Care Financing Administration [Transmittal no. 1528]. Washington, DC: US Government Printing Office.

Meikle M, Wechsler E, Tupper A, Benenson M, Butler J, Mulhall D, Stern G (1979). Comparative trial of volunteer and professional treatments of dysphasia after stroke. British Medical Journal 2: 87–9.

Neisser U (1966). Cognitive Psychology. New York: Appleton-Century-Crofts.

Office of Technology Assessment (1978). Assessing the Efficacy and Safety of Medical Technologies, OTA-H-75. Washington, DC: US Government Printing Office.

Petheram B, Parr S (1998). Diversity in aphasiology: crisis or increasing competence? Aphasiology 12: 435–87.

Ratner NB, Gleason JB (1993). An introduction to psycholinguistics: what do language users know? In Gleason JB, Ratner NB (eds) Psycholinguistics. Fort Worth, TX: Harcourt Brace Jovanovich, pp.1–40.

Robey RR (1994). The efficacy of treatment for aphasic persons: a meta-analysis. Brain and Language 47: 585–608.

Robey RR (1998). A meta-analysis of clinical outcomes in the treatment of aphasia. Journal of Speech, Language, and Hearing Research 41: 172–87.

Robey RR and Schultz MC (1998). A model for conducting clinical outcome research: an adaptation of the standard protocol for use in aphasiology. Aphasiology 12: 787–810.

Rosenbek JC, LaPointe LL, Wertz RT (1989). Aphasia: A Clinical Approach. Austin, TX: pro-ed.

Saffran EM, Schwartz MF, Fink R, Myers J, Martin N (1992). Mapping therapy: an approach to remediating agrammatic sentence comprehension and production. National Institute on Deafness and Other Communication Disorders Monograph 2: 77–90.

Sarno MT (1969). The Functional Communication Profile: Manual of Directions (Rehabilitation Monograph 42). New York: New York University Medical Center, Institute of Rehabilitation Medicine.

Schuell H (1965). The Minnesota Test for Differential Diagnosis of Aphasia. Minneapolis, MN: University of Minnesota Press.

Schuell H, Jenkins JJ, Jimenez-Pabon E (1964). Aphasia in Adults: Diagnosis, Prognosis and Treatment. New York: Hoeber Medical Division, Harper & Row.

Thompson CK, McReynolds L, Vance C (1982). Generative use of locatives in multi-word utterances in agrammatism: a matrix training approach. In Brookshire RH (ed.) Clinical Aphasiology, Volume 8. Minneapolis, MN: BRK, pp.289–97.

Wepman JM (1951). Recovery From Aphasia. New York: Ronald Press.

Wertz RT (1995). Efficacy. In Code C, Muller D (eds) The Treatment of Aphasia: From Theory to Practice. London: Whurr, pp.309–39.

Wertz RT (in press). The role of theory in aphasia therapy: art or science? In Stuss D, Winocur W, Robertson I (eds) Cognitive Neurorehabilitation: A Comprehensive Approach. Cambridge: Cambridge University Press.

Wertz RT, Weiss DG, Aten JL, Brookshire RH, Garcia-Bunuel L, Holland AL, Kurzke JF, LaPointe LL, Milianti FJ, Brannegan R, Greenbaum H, Marshall RC, Vogel D, Carter J, Barnes NS, Goodman R (1986). Comparison of clinic, home, and deferred language treatment for aphasia: a Veterans Administration cooperative study. Archives of Neurology 43: 653–8.

Whurr R, Lorch MP, Nye C (1992). A meta-analysis of studies carried out between 1946 and 1988 concerned with the efficacy of speech and language therapy treatment for aphasic patients. European Journal of Disorders of Communication 27: 1–17.

Whurr R, Lorch M, Nye C (1997) Efficacy of speech and language therapy for aphasia: a meta-analytic review. Neurology Reviews International 1: 9–13.

World Health Organization (1980). The International Classification of Impairments, Disabilities, and Handicaps. Geneva: World Health Organization.

Chapter 2
Recovery of function in aphasia

ILIAS PAPATHANASIOU and RENATA WHURR

Aphasia is defined as a disorder of the comprehension and production of spoken and written language as a result of a brain injury. Recovery from aphasia has interested clinicians for a number of years. Observations of the patterns of clinical recovery have produced many different definitions and descriptions. In this chapter, we will try to synthesize the many different interpretations of recovery of function and show how these different views have influenced the theory and practice of modern aphasia therapy.

The concept of function

Recent advances in our knowledge of how the human brain is organized have resulted in the radical revision of the concept of 'function'. Traditionally, 'function' means the function of a particular tissue, or an organ such as the liver or pancreas. Luria (1973) adopted a different approach and described this concept as a 'complete functional system', with two main features. 'Function', at a system level, is a complex of dynamic structures or combination of centres that formed a 'complete functional system'. The first feature that distinguishes the work of such a system is: 'The presence of a constant (invariant) task, performed by variable (variative) mechanisms, bringing the process to a constant (invariant) result' (Luria, 1973: 28). The second distinguishing feature is the complex composition of the functional system, which always included a series of afferent (adjusting) and efferent (effector) impulses.

This concept of 'function' as a whole functional system is remarkably different from the 'function' of a particular tissue. As the most complex somatic and autonomic processes of the body are organized as 'functional systems' of this type, this concept can be applied to the complex 'functions' of a behaviour. According to Luria (1973), complex mental processes such as language are complex functional systems that are not localized in narrow circumscribed areas of the brain. They take place through the participation of groups of concertedly working brain structures, each of which makes its own particular contribution to the organization of the functional system. He suggested that there were three principal functional systems units of the brain whose participation was necessary for any type of mental activity. These units were described as a unit *for regulating tone or waking*, a unit *for obtaining and storing information* and a unit *for programming, regulating and verifying* mental activity. The three units were hierarchical in structure but worked concertedly, dynamically, systematically and interactively. For a complex mental process to take place they had to work in combination.

The function of communication

Ellis and Beattie (1986) state that 'communication occurs when one organism (the transmitter) encodes information into a signal which passes to another organism (the receiver) which decodes the signal and is capable of responding appropriately'. Applying this definition to the concept of function, as described above, the invariant task is to encode the message, the variable mechanism is how the message is transmitted and the decoding of the message by the receiver is the invariant result. In the 'function of communication', a variety of mental activities, such as attention, comprehension, expression, visual processing, memory and so on, are involved as part of each functional system. The functional system, which regulates tone and waking, is involved in a number of mental activities, such as attention, memory, alertness, comprehension and expression, which enable both participants to be ready for the function to take place. The unit for obtaining and restoring information is involved in mental activities such as memory, comprehension, allocation and storage, and the unit for programming, regulating and verifying mental activity is included in mental activities such as comprehension, expression, semantic processing, memory and so on. Each functional system is therefore contained in different or the same mental activities and they work together and interact dynamically according to the person who communicates, his or her ability to communicate, the situation, the time and other factors that can influence the communication act. However, each of these complex mental activities requires regulation from different parts of the cortical or subcortical areas of both hemispheres of the brain, such as the auditory cortex, the motor cortex, and subcortical areas such as the basal ganglia, thalamus and insula. Therefore, in order to understand the 'function of communication', its impairment and recovery, we have to understand how all the principal functional brain units work concertedly, their interactions during their contribution, and the nature of the cerebral mechanisms involved in a mental activity.

The function of language in aphasia

Language is a widely used term, which has accumulated divergent conno-
tations, many of which are not germane to the discussion of aphasia
(Whurr, 1982). What is largely agreed on is that aphasia is a central
language disorder which has repercussions for all modalities of language
(speaking, understanding, reading and writing). The earliest attempt to
consider linguistic description as the basis for studying aphasia was by the
neurologist Sir Henry Head (1926), who used the terms verbal, syntactic,
semantic and nominal in his description of a patient (see Whurr, 1982).
In 1961, Wepman and Jones identified three types of aphasia: pragmatic,
syntactic and semantic, but there was lack of cohesion in their descriptive
system. As a linguist, Roman Jakobson (1956) made the first and major
contribution to the linguistic study of aphasia. He described aphasic
disorders as those of a combination or contiguity of linguistic units, and
as those disorders of selection or similarity. This was based on his distinction between the message – a combination of constituent parts
(sentences, words, phonemes, and so on) – and the code – a combination
of all possible constituents. His classification was criticized as basic and
simple, but he introduced the concept of studying the different linguistic
levels and linguistic function in a systematic way. This concept became
the basis of the functional working definition of language in terms of how
language is processed in normal human beings. More recently, Westbury
(1998) comments that a functional definition of language will have a
hierarchical structured definition, but some aspects of language work
across all modalities, with their bimodal properties. Looking at the hierarchical structure, at the top level of classification there is a distinction
between the two main language modalities: spoken and written
language. In each of these modalities, language breaks down into input
and output functions, although this distinction is more complex than it
seems. The input and output classes may be broken into two subhierar-
chies. In both classes, one subhierarchy is linked to the semantic
modality. The second subhierarchy consists of a set of components,
which function to access the elements of language, defined by the hierarchical deconstruction of the input and output streams relevant to that
modality. In the written modality, these are the sentences, words and
letters, and in the auditory modality they are sentences, words and
phonemes. Interaction takes place between these modalities, and some
of the components can function independently or serve the special role
of translating between input and output or written and oral modalities.
Aspects of language with bimodal properties, such as affixes, low-
frequency words and abstract words are not organized in this hierarchical
structure but influence the way the hierarchies are accessed and subsequently how language functions. In order to complete the above
concepts of the linguistic function, we have to consider the environment
in which that function takes place and the behaviours associated with it.

Language is a means of communication, thus any functional linguistic system must underpin the function of communication. The principles underlying the dynamic organization of language and communication are regulated by different cortical and subcortical brain functional units. Changes in the communicative behaviour of people with acquired aphasia are in essence the result of changes in the cellular and neuronal organization of the brain.

The concepts of plasticity and recovery

In aphasia, the evolution and recovery of language and communication involve alteration in the brain as a result of cellular, physiological, structural and behavioural changes. These changes can be considered at two different levels, the micro level (cellular/neural level) and the macro level (system/behavioural level).

What is plasticity?

According to Kolb (1995), plasticity is considered to be the brain's capacity to change at either micro level (cellular/network level), which is known as neural plasticity, or macro level (behavioural/system level), known as behavioural plasticity, allowing it to respond to environmental changes or changes in the organism itself. The underlying mechanisms of neural plasticity are multiple and they include biochemical, physiological, structural and functional changes. The consequences of these changes, which express themselves in behavioural plasticity, are likewise multiple. Plasticity allows the brain to learn new behaviours and skills. At the same time, the behaviour itself can alter the brain, which in turn facilitates the behaviour. Thus, plasticity results from alterations in behaviour, and vice versa. Brain damage results in behaviour changes and these in turn produce changes in the brain. Frackowiack (1997) defines plasticity, using a more empirical functional approach based more at the macro systemic level, as the changes of neural function over time or, in other words, the adaptation of activity with repeated behaviour or following injury. Thus, plasticity takes place because of the alterations of distributed patterns of normal task-associated brain activity that accompany action, perception and cognition and that compensate impaired function from disease or brain injury.

What is recovery?

In the injured brain, these behavioural changes of function are described by Brandt et al. (1997) in terms of what we usually refer to as recovery. The term recovery is often used as a synonym for other terms referring to behavioural changes such as restoration, reorganization, compensation, habituation, restitution, substitution, learning and so on.

The recovery, in terms of description, is independent of the underlying mechanisms or structural changes at a micro level as it refers to behaviours and functional systems at a macro level. However, there is an interaction between the two levels in terms of direction, time and the mechanisms by which they occur.

Timescale and patterns of recovery

The evolution of recovery after brain injury follows a general pattern. Immediately after the trauma there is a short period of shock in which many functions are depressed. These are followed by a period of rapid recovery, which takes place over a few hours or days, and then a steady improvement over several weeks which gradually ceases as the months and years go by. According to Powell (1981), three different plastic neuronal mechanisms are relevant to the timescale of the recovery process (see Figure 2.1). First, there is the mechanism of physical repair, which is important during the initial days as the wound and body heals, scar tissue forms and the disturbed physiological functions revert to normal. Second, there are mechanisms that adapt to the deficit by reorganizing the way the person behaves or restructuring neural processing to take advantage of intact areas. Such adaptation is apparent from the beginning and is likely to peak as the person learns about the nature of the deficit; it will then decline in importance as the limits of the reshuffling are reached. Finally, there are new learning mechanisms which govern the extent to which the person can be retrained to perform a skill and to adapt to his or her loss.

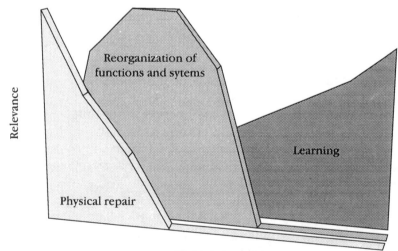

Figure 2.1: The evolution of the different mechanisms for the recovery of function since injury.

Kolb (1995) describes the timescale of the course of recovery using a more reductionist approach to the original function, and identifies three possible outcomes. Initially, there may be compensation resulting from the adaptation to the loss. This could reflect a change in strategy, or represent the substitution of a new behaviour for the lost one. A second outcome might be a partial restitution of the original behaviour, which could reflect recovery from a non-specific effect of the injury or might reflect the genuine return of the function. Third, there could be a complete restitution of the original behaviour. This happens as the structural properties of the brain allow plastic changes to take place, which allow recovery to occur. However, the structural properties of the brain are important to its function and any permanent injury will affect function permanently. So, a function returning completely and truly to its original form can be described only in theoretical and not in clinical terms. Therefore, 'recovery' must be evaluated as partial recovery of function and partial substitution or, in more functional terms, as less behavioural loss.

Powell (1981) suggests that the complexity of the recovery process cannot be overstated. Function can follow various courses of recovery because of the differential physiological and structural organization. Specific mechanisms of recovery will be applicable to some functions and irrelevant to others. There are also individual differences in cerebral organization that will influence recovery, and individual differences when it comes to strategic learning. Thus, recovery is a multiple mechanism, across time, across functions and across people themselves. Overall, Powell describes five different courses of recovery of function:

- *Composite or general curve of recovery*: this refers to immediate loss of efficiency of function followed by progressively less rapid recovery.
- *Unaffected function*: initial loss of function due to general trauma and immediate return to former level, when the lesion is not a site critical for this function.
- *Temporarily suppressed function*: the loss of function recovers in days or weeks, for example, there is often a rapid recovery of speech after a stroke.
- *Loss of function*: This loss is followed by the gradual return and relearning of function using compensatory strategies, with some observable residual deficit.
- *Loss of unrecoverable function*: this loss remains as a severe deficit.

Powell (1981) suggests that once the physiological repair and restitution has taken place and the bounds of the pre-existing structure or potential have been reached, the organism may still be impaired in its functioning. Then, the only way that an organism can make progress is to use strategies of task solution that bypass the lesion site and use only healthy brain and intact functions. The fact of using new strategies may itself prompt further physiological changes (for example, new connections are encouraged in specific directions) or even encourage further structural changes (such as 'helping' an area to take on a new function). Keefe (1995) suggests that, if we wed our knowledge of the changes that occur in the brain in response to behavioural events and the neural mechanisms that underlie them with our understanding of the nature of the functions of language and communication in the brain and how it is disrupted by nervous system injury, then the behaviour intervention that we use to treat aphasia may be more effective. Therefore, for the most effective treatment of a dysfunction arising from an organic lesion, such as the dysfunction of language and communication observed in aphasia, we need not only psychological analysis of the deficits based on the hierarchical cognitive processing approach, but also a detailed neuropsychological analysis that reflects the organic brain structures of the functional system that is disturbed.

The relationship of recovery and plasticity

To understand how the recovery of language and communication takes place, we have to consider all the mechanisms involved in neural and behavioural plasticity. The mechanisms of neural plasticity can be classified as biochemical/physiological at a cellular level, structural at the brain structure level and behavioural at the system network level. This classification is rather arbitrary as there is a dynamic interaction among the levels, and mechanisms that might take place at one level may reflect and present changes at a different level. Kolb (1995) states the properties of this brain–behaviour dynamic interactive relation, which makes brain plastic and subsequently alter its expression in the form of behaviours, as:

- Behavioural states and mind states correspond to brain states
- The structural properties of the brain are important in understanding its function
- Plasticity is a property of the synapse
- Behavioural plasticity results from the summation of plasticity of individual neurones
- Specific mechanisms of plasticity are likely to underlie more than one form of behavioural change
- The cortex is the most likely candidate for neural plasticity
- Behaviour is difficult to study as molecules.

In contrast, Powell (1981) states the properties of the language–brain dynamic relation from the other direction of how a behaviour can make the brain plastic, as:

- A cognitive capacity such as language may have more than one mode of expression
- Superficially similar or functionally equivalent material may be analysed or stored in distinct areas of the brain
- In the damaged brain, intact areas can become involved in attempting to perform the lost function
- Language tasks activate the right hemisphere as well as the left
- Language, in a normal left-hemisphere-dominant individual, has not been solely in the left hemisphere
- Normal language uses certain pathways, but others may exist which, although they are not normally used, may come into play when primary routes are damaged.

In the following sections we will describe these mechanisms from the neuronal to behavioural levels.

Biochemical and physiological mechanisms of recovery of function

Injury in the brain following a stroke or other forms of damage produces both primary and secondary changes. The primary changes evolve from the first hours up to a number of days and then they will become static, but the secondary changes continue to evolve over time and develop as a consequence of the primary damage (Keefe, 1995). Importantly, because these processes develop over a longer timescale than the primary changes associated with the lesion, the organization and function of the brain a few days after the injury will be different from that a few weeks after the injury. Secondary changes are the processes that determine and contribute to the behavioural recovery and the residual deficits observed, and not, as was thought traditionally, the site of lesion (Powell, 1981; Keefe, 1995).

The immediate changes that happen following the lesion can be classified as primary (directly related to the trauma area) and secondary (indirectly, as a consequence of the primary changes). (Powell, 1981; Keefe, 1995). The primary changes are immediate necrosis, signs of inflammation in the cell, retrograde cell degeneration proximal to the lesion, and anterograde cell degeneration distal to the lesion within a week of the trauma. The indirect changes are: *transneuronal degeneration*, in which areas receiving neural input from, or providing input to, the infarcted area degenerate due to the loss of connections; *denervation supersensitivity*, in which neurones that have lost most of their input from the infarcted area become increasingly sensitive to any residual input received from that area; *development of diaschisis*, in which injury to a certain area will temporarily inhibit connected non-injured areas remote from the infarcted tissue but yet functionally connected to it; *vascular disruption*, which will result in ischaemia; and *collateral sprouting*, in which axons from nearby neurones grow new synaptic contacts on sites vacated by the lesioned cells.

As we have described above, these secondary changes have a longer timescale and contribute to behavioural recovery and highlight the plasticity which takes place in the adult brain. These plastic changes take place via different physiological mechanisms of recovery of function, which can be summarized as:

* *Regenerative sprouting* (Powell, 1981): This regeneration concerns changes in the severed neurone. The impaired axon regenerates fibres from other branches of the lesioned axon that are capable of forming a functional network, where they form working synapses proximal to the area of destruction, which will pass on an impulse to another neurone.
* *Collateral regenerative sprouting* (Powell, 1981; Keefe, 1995): This regeneration concerns growth in other non-lesioned cells. These cells grow new synaptic connections that are connected to the synaptic areas that are not functioning after the lesion. These new connections may enable the affected site to function 'normally' again by providing its lost input.
* *Relatively ineffective synapses* (Powell, 1981): This concept concerns the possibility that what seems to be the formation of new connections may in fact be the 'waking up' of pre-existing connections that were originally ineffective for this function and overshadowed by the main connections of the cell.
* *Denervation sensitivity* (Powell, 1981; Keefe, 1995): After the injury the cell shows a lower response threshold to any remaining afferent fibres. Subsequently, the remaining fibres that use the same neurotransmitters as the lesioned fibres will cause a larger effect in the recipient cell, so that, although the number of afferents might be reduced, they have the same enervating effect as the full complement.
* *Long-term potentiation (LTP)* (Keefe, 1995; Leonard, 1998): LTP is the neural explanation for learning and memory. It is a rapidly induced and sustained increase in the efficiency of neural transmission at a given synapse between the stimulating axon and its post-synaptic cell. So, the synapse that is highly active, secondary to increased stimulation of input, will exhibit LTP and thus enhanced activity. This neural mechanism can cause long-term changes in the transmission of a synapse, and subsequently to the functional systems related to this synapse.

The exact role of the above physiological mechanisms in the recovery of function in clinical terms may need further explanation, as the interaction between them is not yet understood and neither is their link to specific behavioural changes. At the interactional level, some of them may contradict others: for example, the inhibitory character of the diaschisis may not facilitate the collateral sprouting. However, as these mechanisms have been observed in experimental situations, the challenge is to find the correlations between neuronal and behavioural changes. Great insight into this challenge is provided by the use of pharmacological agents to facilitate and enhance recovery of function. Adequate cognitive function requires a relatively high level of neurochemical capacity (Blomert, 1998). Functional (metabolic) 'lesions' may represent depressed levels of neurotransmitters and thus form the basis of many processing limitations. Luria et al. (1969) used a combination of pharmacological and behavioural treatment for seemingly permanent disorders and showed significant behavioural improvement by boosting the level of the neurotransmitter acetylcholine. Also, recently, Huber et al. (1997) showed the beneficial effects of the drug piracetam when it was used in a chronic aphasic patient in combination with systematic language training. Walker-Batson et al. (1996) have shown that the administration of amphetamine accelerates recovery from aphasia. These findings might suggest that pharmacological and/or stimulation treatment preceding training may sufficiently alter neurochemical activity levels to make improvements and enhance the recovery process.

Structural mechanisms of recovery of function

The physiological mechanisms discussed refer to what happens at the cellular level to repair affected connections. However, evidence of plasticity is available not only from examination of the function of the synapse but also from examination of the brain's molar structure as a whole (Keefe, 1995). Traditionally, various theories of structural mechanisms have been developed to provide an explanation for the reappearance of a 'lost' function following brain lesion (Blomert, 1998). However, today, neuroscientists have established that the brain responds to damage by triggering complex processes that take place over long periods of time and that produce changes throughout the entire nervous system (Stein and Glazier, 1992). But the early theoretical accounts still provide a framework for current research. These theories are described as:

- *The resolution or regression of diaschisis* (Powell, 1981; Cappa, 1998): The initial diaschisis, which is considered to be an initial protective mechanism of the brain to the injury, like any other form of inhibition, tends to extinguish or disappear, allowing several centre of the brain to be able to function again. According to Luria (1963), there is an established pattern of recovery from diaschisis, with physical and functional thresholds changing first, followed by thresholds of subjective sensation.

- *Mass action theory*, also known as *equipotentiality* (Powell, 1981; Leonard, 1998): This theory states that any part of the brain is capable of subserving any function, and that most functions are represented all over the cortex. This suggests that a function lost secondary to damage to a specific region of the nervous system can be mediated by a surviving structure or pathway.
- *Redundancy* (Powell, 1981; Blomert, 1998): The concept of redundancy can refer to either the level of neural processing or the task level. At the neural processing level, redundancy theory assumes that uninjured neurones in the damaged area function as spare systems that can compensate for those that are non-functional. At a task level, it is assumed that a task might carry multiple cues, which are transmitted neurally. In the case that some of the cues become redundant, the task might still be completed by using compensatory strategies.
- *Vicarious function theory* (Blomert, 1998; Leonard, 1998): This theory suggests that another area of the brain, not previously involved in a particular function, takes over the function of the damaged areas. This might involve synapses that originally had a very weak input into the system, which, after damage, becomes the strongest available remaining input.
- *Substitution theory* (Powell, 1981; Leonard, 1998): This proposes that a behaviour can be performed by a different mechanism than that which originally controlled the behaviour. In other words, the end is achieved by different means, served by regions that were not involved before and now become active.
- *Functional takeover* (Cappa, 1998): In the case of lateralized functions such as language, this theory suggests that functions can be taken over by the undamaged contralateral hemisphere. This is considered to be the 'unmasking' of a pre-existent functional commitment, inhibited by the left hemisphere (Moscovitch, 1977). Another possibility is that the functional takeover is the result of reorganization in the same hemisphere, as it is described in the vicarious function theory.

The role of the mechanisms proposed by these theories in the recovery of function is still controversial, as the mechanisms of recovery do not relate to these theories (Stein and Glazier, 1992). The gap between theories and mechanisms may be diminished by the technological advances that are the bases of current research.

What is the evidence for structural mechanisms involved in recovery of function?

Today, advances in laboratory data from animal studies, brain imaging techniques and neurophysiological techniques and measures provide some empirical evidence for structural mechanisms involved in the recovery of function.

Keefe (1995) gives an account of animal studies that indicate changes in the structure of the nervous system. These changes are described as an increase in the dendritic branching and functional reorganization of the cortical maps. First, dendritic branching is influenced by rich, environmentally stimulating tasks, which indicates that learning- or environment-induced changes in cortical structure are highly associated with the specific task demands. Also, dendritic branching of neurones is influenced by central nervous system damage. In animal studies, functional reorganization of the cortical maps is observed following behavioural intervention and is associated with changes in both the ipsilateral and contralateral areas adjacent to the lesioned brain regions. However, these changes in the nervous system network could be limited by the nature and extent of the existing sensory connections, and their association to primary and secondary cortical areas. Similar mechanisms of functional reorganization are observed under the influence of stimulating environmental tasks (Keefe, 1995). Also, similar cortical reorganization in animals, as reflected in alterations in cortical maps, is seen following cortical injury. At the site of the lesion, the remaining receptive field-size neurones become larger and the lesion affects more distant cortical areas, in particular the secondary areas of representation that are connected to long-term recovery of function. The parameters determining the nature of this aspect of reorganization are not known.

The brain-imaging studies provide dynamic and structural information. Dynamic information is obtained by positron emission tomography (PET), which involves measures of regional cerebral blood flow and glucose metabolism. Structural information is provided by functional magnetic resonance imaging (fMRI) studies. Cappa (1998) gives an account of the study of the mechanism of diaschisis and its regression using PET. The presence of diaschisis has been related to the severity of the clinical picture following the acute period after the lesion (Cappa, 1998). In a series of studies, Metter et al. (1992) assessed regional cerebral metabolic abnormalities in structurally affected and unaffected areas in aphasic patients. They found a significant positive correlation between changes in left and right temporoparietal glucose metabolism and changes in auditory comprehension. Heis et al. (1993) reported that the level of glucose metabolism in the left hemisphere outside the infarcted area in the acute stage was the best predictor of recovery of auditory comprehension after 4 months, suggesting the importance of intrahemispheric diaschisis in the recovery of function. Also, in the same study, they reported that in a subgroup of mildly aphasic patients, metabolic values in the infarcted temporoparietal area, left Broca's area and contralateral mirror to the lesion area were predictive of the recovery of auditory comprehension, which indicates the possibility of extensive bilateral contribution of brain areas to the recovery of function.

Cappa et al. (1997) examined the regression of functional deactivation during the recovery of lesion in the cortical areas of language by measuring the regional glucose metabolism. The study showed that even 6 months post-onset, metabolic depression, which correlates with functional deactivation, was present in structurally unaffected areas both ipsilateral and contralateral to lesion site. In addition, an association was found between the regression of deactivation in the unaffected areas connected with the lesion site and the recovery observed. Cortical functional reorganization in both hemispheres has been reported in a number of PET studies investigating the regional cerebral activation in recovered and non-recovered aphasics while they were engaged in linguistic and non-linguistic tasks, which allows more direct investigation of functional recovery after acute damage. Wellio et al. (1995) studied a group of partially recovered Wernicke's aphasics using PET scans, and showed a significant recruitment of frontal and temporal areas of the right hemisphere, mirroring the left hemispheric areas that were activated in the normal subjects. Buckner et al. (1996) also reported right lateralized prefrontal response in a patient during a word-stem completion task, suggesting recruitment of a brain compensatory pathway. Frackowiak (1997) reports two further studies of language recovery in aphasic patients compared with normals, one investigating non-word repetition and verb generation and the other investigating reading. Frackowiak observed bilateral language activation not only in the recovered subjects, but also in the controls when they were viewing words, which indicates the contribution of the right hemisphere in some language functions. In some subjects, recovery of function was related to peri-infarct activation, with no activation of the right hemisphere. Following the findings of these studies, it is suggested that recovery of language depends on the viability of peri-infarct tissue and the premorbid lateralization of language. Overall, these findings provide considerable evidence that there are long-lasting changes in the patterns of cerebral activation, which are related to clinically observable behavioural changes.

Further evidence of the mechanisms of recovery and plasticity have started to emerge from the increased use of non-invasive neurophysiological techniques not only in experimental but also in clinical studies. Transcranial magnetic stimulation (TMS) is a painless technique for stimulating the brain through the scalp and provides insight into the timing of information processing in the neuronal system. It can induce a positive effect or disrupt a neural function by magnetic stimulation of the scalp. TMS also provides cortical maps of neuronal functions and can highlight specific pathways and connections in a functional system

(Pascual-Leone and Meador, 1998). Epstein (1998), in an overview of the current experimental use of TMS in language function, reports that TMS is used to interfere with language expression, comprehension and verbal recall by creating temporarily reversible lesions, or to facilitate language-related functions and motor function through language. Topper et al. (1998) reported facilitation in a picture-naming task by focal TMS on Wernicke's area. Tokimura et al. (1996) reported that reading aloud may increase excitability of the motor hand area in the dominant hemisphere. Cohen et al. (1998) described the different ways in which TMS can be used to identify patterns of reorganization of function, the mechanisms involved in cortical plasticity and the relevance of these patterns to behavioural changes. Papathanasiou et al. (in preparation) used TMS to investigate the recovery of the function of writing in aphasic hemiplegic patients and reported on the contribution of pathways contralateral and ipsilateral to the site of lesion.

Another technique for studying the functional system of language is that of magnetoencephalography, which allows spatial localization of the neuronal pools with an extremely high time resolution (Rossini et al., 1998). Simos et al. (1998) used this technique to study the functional cerebral laterality of language on normal subjects using a semantic-matching and a tone-matching tasks. They reported that this technique can be used for laterality assessment.

The development and availability of these tools, and the new evidence provided in both experimental and clinical studies, should contribute to our improved understanding of the patterns, mechanisms and functional relevance of cortical plasticity. These developments should lead to the design of effective strategies to enhance brain plasticity in a beneficial way and thus boost the recovery of functional systems after brain injury.

Behavioural mechanisms in recovery of function

The behavioural mechanisms of recovery of function refer to the capacity of the brain to recover function beyond the limitations of the physiological and structural repair (Powell, 1981). Behavioural changes may in themselves trigger or even encourage further physiological and structural changes. These physiological and structural changes at the micro level may be manipulated at the macro behavioural level in terms of direction, type and time of change, both spontaneously or by specific intervention (Cappa, 1998).

The behavioural mechanisms of recovery of function are:

- *Restitution–restoration–reactivation* (Huber, Springer and Willmes, 1993; Lesser and Milroy, 1993; Carlomagno and Iavarone, 1995; Blomert, 1998): These three terms, which are often used interchangeably in the literature, refer to the same mechanism. The mechanism applies to the total return of the function by using means in the same functional system similar to those in the pre-lesion situation. Huber et al. (1993) describe direct stimulation, indirect stimulation and deblocking as methods of treatment to enhance the evolution of temporarily impaired language function. They suggest that a detailed analysis of task demands in terms of input, output and central processing in the impaired functional system is important to determine the stimulus task used in therapy.

- *Reorganization or reconstitution or substitution within a functional system* (Howard and Hatfield, 1987; Lesser and Milroy, 1993; Edmundson and McIntosh, 1995): This mechanism, originally described by Luria, suggests that within a functional system it is possible to reroute parts of the function without excluding the whole functional system. This can be accomplished by 'filling in the missing link' of the functional system. The new route is different from the one that would normally be used, but the end result is the same. Bruce and Howard (1987) describe a treatment approach where word-finding problems were overcome with the use of a self-induced strategy of phonemic cueing. This strategy provided access to the phonological form of the word by using knowledge about grapheme–phoneme conversion rules. The grapheme–phoneme conversion was facilitated by teaching patients with the aid of a computer. Patients had to select the first letter of the target word on the computer keyboard, listen to the computer-generated phonemic cue and then attempt to produce it.

- *Relearning* (Howard and Hatfield, 1987; Edmundson and McIntosh, 1995): This mechanism implies the ability to use strategies to relearn lost items or information, or to re-establish lost rules or procedures in a functional system. De Partz (1986) reports using this mechanism in therapy to teach an aphasic patient to relearn the phoneme–grapheme conversion orthographic rules of reading; for example, how the pronunciation of different consonants changes in the context of different vowels.

- *Facilitation* (Howard and Hatfield, 1987; Edmundson and McIntosh, 1995): This mechanism, usually employed as a therapy strategy, indicates when the deficit is that of an access procedure. So, this mechanism enables access or improved access to intact information in a functional system. Marshall et al. (1990) use this mechanism in the therapy of a patient with difficulties accessing his speech output lexicon, although his semantic processing, comprehension of word pictures, and reading aloud of regular and irregular words were relatively intact. The strategy used aimed to reinforce links between the semantic representations and the phonological output representations, and thus improve access to the speech output lexicon.

- *Functional substitution, functional reorganization or functional compensation* (Powell, 1981; Lesser and Milroy, 1993; Carlomagno and Iavarone, 1995; Blomert, 1998): This refers to the mechanism that acts when the original function cannot recover in its original functional system. Then, a different functional system from intact areas of the brain can substitute for the loss and limitations of the original function, in order to complete the task for which the original functional system was responsible. So, this mechanism is more one of adaptation than the actual recovery of function since no attempt is made to restore the original function and there is no reason to believe it is a real recovery. Clear illustrations of this mechanism are the use of lip-reading in acquired deafness; the use of gestures, computers or other devices as the main means of communication following loss of speech in aphasic patients; and the use of the left hand for writing when the right hand is paralysed in aphasic hemiplegic patients.
- *Connectionism* (Small, 1994): The recently developed connectionist model, which focuses on the interplay of a computational localized model, the formal specification of the computational process, behavioural mechanisms, and anatomical-physiological structures, is a contender in the study of language disorders. This approach has yet to be tried and tested.

The above behavioural mechanisms have been described more as part of the recovery of the function of language and might not reflect the function of communication from a holistic perspective. In order to examine the recovery of the function of communication, we should consider the communication strategies adopted by patients and carers through alterations in behaviour or the context and environment in which the behaviour occurs. These strategies, which may arise from different functional systems of mental activities and the behavioural mechanisms associated with them accumulating and interacting together, aim to enable the patient to be an 'effective' communicator in his or her environment.

Ideally, we should look at the interactive mechanisms of multiple systems in the recovery process and not just consider a purely hierarchical approach. To do this ignores the social and interactive dimensions that are important aspects of communication. If we look at the behavioural mechanisms of language recovery, resulting from structural and biological mechanisms at a micro level, the same structural and biological mechanisms are responsible not only for the recovery of the function of language but also for the recovery of other mental activities. We could assume that the same basic behavioural mechanisms such as relearning, facilitation and reorganization are used across all functional systems and are responsible for the recovery of the function of communication.

Reconceptualizing aphasia and aphasia therapy

Understanding these intricate mechanisms of recovery of function has implications for our conceptualization of aphasia and aphasia therapy. Aphasia is considered to be a dysfunction of the functional system of language and communication due to an organic neurological lesion. This dysfunction is evident at a central cognitive level, is of neurological origin and results in impairments in both linguistic and communication behaviours. The course of recovery depends on a spectrum of biochemical, physiological, structural and behavioural mechanisms, which need to be in place to promote recovery. The fundamental question is how these mechanisms can be manipulated to enable the person to achieve his full communicative potential. But, for simple question like this, the answer is rather complicated.

Some of the mechanisms follow a timescale of evolution, such as diaschisis, and can be maladaptive in the recovery of the functional system. The structural properties of these mechanisms will have existed prior to injury and can only be considered as background potentials, which may or may not be activated by functional changes.

In clinical practice, therapists may analyse and intervene only at the behavioural level, without considering the underlying neuronal organization. The structural properties of neuronal organization may be manipulated in a more efficient way. Keefe (1995) emphasizes the importance of the neuronal organization of the mechanisms that have implications for aphasia therapy. It is suggested that long-term potentiation (LTP) could be the neuronal mechanism underlying the effects of intense stimulation therapies, with the input given from the impaired or intact modality to a given population of neurones enhancing the effectiveness of the synapses remaining from the impaired modality. Also, the cortical reorganization as result of behavioural and environmental influence may be relevant to the refinement and development of therapy approaches, to determine the type, intensity and frequency of input needed to obtain behavioural reorganization, and explore the impact of such therapy approaches on cortical reorganization. Overall, we have to understand the implications of these mechanisms for treatment by considering three important aspects of their role in the recovery of function. First, we have to estimate the capacity of the mechanism to explain why a lesion may not lead to any observable consequence. Second, we need to determine the relevance of each mechanism to the recovery of function along a timescale. Finally, we need to assess how likely it is that each mechanism might be manipulated through behavioural intervention in therapy in such a way that its evolution will not have any harmful effects.

Powell (1981) described the timescale of the different plastic neuronal mechanisms that are relevant to the recovery process and subsequently to the evolution of aphasia (see Figure 2.1). Consequently, principles and methods of aphasia therapy vary according to the patient's phase of recovery. Huber et al. (1993) described three phases of aphasia therapy: activation, symptom-specific training and consolidation. These phases could correspond directly to the mechanism of physical repair observed in the first days, to the mechanism of adapting to the deficit and to the learning mechanism as described by Powell (1981). Huber at al. (1993) also suggest that all phases of aphasia therapy should be accompanied by family support and psychosocial support for the patient, as the clinical regimen should always comprise both therapy for aphasia and therapy for the aphasic person. During the period of activation the therapy goals should be to enhance the evolution of temporarily impaired language functions. So, therapy should focus on those parts of the functional system that are temporarily suppressed or temporarily lost their efficiency. The therapeutic overall goal during this acute phase is to activate the patient by all available means to respond communicatively as appropriately as possible. Techniques such as direct stimulation, indirect stimulation and deblocking are used, which enable behavioural mechanisms in a functional system to recover.

The symptom-specific training starts when the initial physical repair has been completed. At this stage, it is possible to evaluate extensively the loss of the functional abilities of the aphasic person. Huber (1992) suggests that therapy should aim for the relearning of degraded linguistic knowledge, the reactivation of impaired linguistic modalities, and the relearning of compensatory linguistic strategies. However, the issue of whether therapy should be focused on the treatment of specific deficits of the impaired modalities or the practice and use of the residual deficient skills in relation to the evolution of recovery, remains unclear. But it is assumed that both these approaches, which represent the substitution and functional compensation mechanisms respectively, are responsible for the functional recovery of the system. Therapy approaches applied at this stage are the language-oriented learning approaches such as those looking at linguistic structures, linguistic modalities, linguistic strategies, cognitive models of language processing, cognitive capacity processing and so on.

The final phase is consolidation, where the learning mechanisms are used to complement and maintain the linguistic skills learned in the previous phase, to enhance them and transfer them to everyday communicative situations (Huber et al., 1993). During this phase, the functional system of language and communication is used at its full capacity, with support from other functional systems, to enable the person to achieve communicative effectiveness. Therapeutic techniques used are those of role playing, PACE therapy, conversation coaching, teaching carers communicative strategies, use of gestures or other non-verbal strategies, and so on. According to Powell (1981), the timescale and the evolution of these phases in aphasia in relation to the underpinning mechanisms of the recovery function depend on many factors: the variables of the tasks used in therapy; patient parameters such as age, occupation, educational background and so on; the patient's motivation to participate; and the environment in which therapy takes place.

Ideally, in clinical practice, what is required is a detailed analysis of the communication task in terms of input, output and central processing across the impaired functional system. In therapy, what is needed is to determine the stimulus task precisely to activate and promote the neurodynamics underlying the function.

In conclusion, it is important to assess the contribution and the relationship of all the mechanisms involved to the changes observed during recovery. In other words, we still need more empirical evidence in order to formulate a link between the analysis of performance of a functional system, the neurophysiology of brain functions and the evolution of aphasia. Such links will enable us to design therapy and deliver it in a more efficient way.

References

Blomert L (1998). Recovery from language disorders: interactions between brain and rehabilitation. In Stemmer B, Whitaker HA (eds) Handbook of Neurolinguistics. San Diego, CA: Academic Press, pp.548–59.

Brandt T, Strupp M, Arbusow V, Dieringer N (1997). Plasticity of the vestibular system: central compensation and sensory substitution for vestibular deficits. In Freund HJ, Sbel BA, Witte OW (eds) Advances in Neorology : Brain Plasticity, Volume 73. Philadelphia, PA: Lippincott-Raven, pp.297–309.

Bruce C, Howard D (1987). Computer-generated phonemic cues: an effective aid for naming in aphasia. British Journal of Communication Disorders 22: 191–201.

Buckner RL, Corbetta M, Scatz J, Raichle ME, Petersen SE (1996). Preserved speech abilities and compensation following prefrontal damage. Proceedings of the National Academy of Science, USA 93: 1249–53.

Cappa SF (1998). Spontaneous recovery in aphasia. In Stemmer B, Whitaker HA (eds) Handbook of Neurolinguistics. San Diego, CA: Academic Press, pp.536–47.

Cappa SF, Perani D, Grassi F, Bressi S, Alberoni M, Franceschi M, Bettinardi V, Todde S, Fazio E (1997). A PET follow up study of recovery after stroke in acute aphasics. Brain and Language 56: 55–67.

Carlomagno S, Iavarone A (1995). Writing rehabilitation in aphasic patients. In Code C, Muller D (eds) Treatment of Aphasia: From Theory to Practice. London: Whurr, pp.201–22.

Cohen LG, Ziemann U, Chen R, Classen J, Hallet M, Gerloff C, Butefisch C (1998). Studies of neuroplasticity with transcranial magnetic stimulation. Journal of Clinical Neurophysiology 15(4): 305–24.

De Partz MP (1986). Re-education of a deep dyslexic patient: rationale of the methods and results. Cognitive Neuropsychology 3: 149–77.

Edmundson A, McIntosh J (1995). Cognitive neuropsychology and aphasia therapy: putting the theory into practice. In Code C, Muller D (eds) Treatment of Aphasia: From Theory to Practice. London: Whurr, pp.137–63.

Ellis A, Beattie G (1986). The Psychology of Language and Communication. London: Lawrence Erlbaum.

Epstein C (1998). Transcranial magnetic stimulation: language function. Journal of Clinical Neurophysiology 15(4): 325–32.

Frackowiack RSJ (1997). The cerebral basis of functional recovery. In Frackowiack RSJ, Friston KJ, Frith CD, Dolan RJ, Mazziotta JC (eds) Human Brain Function. London: Academic Press, pp.275–99.

Heis WD, Kessler J, Karbe H, Fink GR, Pawlik G (1993). Cerebral glucose metabolism as a predictor of recovery from aphasia in ischaemic stroke. Archives of Neurology 50: 958–64.

Howard D, Hatfield F (1987). Aphasia Therapy: Historical and Contemporary Issues. London: Lawrence Erlbaum.

Huber W (1992). Therapy of aphasia: comparison of various approaches. In Steinbuche NV, von Cramon DY, Poppel E (eds) Neuropsychological Rehabilitation. Heidelberg: Springer, pp.242–56.

Huber W, Springer L, Willmes K (1993). Approaches to aphasia therapy in Aachen. In Holland AL, Forbes MM (eds) Aphasia Treatment – World Perspectives. San Diego, CA: Singular, pp.55–86.

Huber W, Willmes K, Poeck K, Van Vleymen B, Deberdt W (1997). Piracetam as an adjuvant to language therapy for aphasia: a randomized double-blind placebo-controlled pilot study. Archives of Physical Medicine and Rehabilitation 78: 245–50.

Jakobson R (1956). Two aspects of language and two types of aphasic disturbance. In Jakobson R, Halle M (eds) Fundamentals of Language. The Hague: Mouton, pp.235–68.

Keefe K (1995). Applying basic neurosciences to aphasia therapy: what the animal studies are telling us. American Journal of Speech–Language Pathology 4: 88–93.

Kolb B (1995). Brain Plasticity and Behavior. Mahwah, NJ: Lawrence Erlbaum.

Leonard CT (1998). The Neuroscience of Human Movement. St Louis, MO: Mosby.

Lesser R, Milroy L (1993). Linguistics and Aphasia: Psycholinguistic and Pragmatic Aspects of Intervention. London: Longman.

Luria A (1963). Restoration of Function after Brain Injury. London: Pergamon Press.

Luria A (1973). The Working Brain. Harmondsworth: Penguin.

Luria AR, Naydin VL, Tsvetkota LS, Vinarskaya EN (1969). Restoration of higher cortical function following local brain damage. In Vinken PJ, Bruyn GW (eds) Handbook of Clinical Neurology, Volume 3. Amsterdam: North Holland, pp.368–433.

Marshall J, Pound C, White-Thomson M, Pring T (1990). The use of picture/word matching tasks to assist word retrieval in aphasic patients. Aphasiology 4: 167–84.

Metter EJ, Jackson CA, Kempler D, Hanson WR (1992). Temporoparietal cortex and the recovery of language comprehension in aphasia. Aphasiology 6: 349–58.

Moscovitch M (1977). The development of lateralisation of language and its relation to cognitive and linguistic development: a review of some theoretical speculations. In Segalowitz SJ, Gruber FA (eds) Language Development and Neurological Theory. New York: Academic Press, pp.193–211.

Papathanasiou I, Whurr R, Jahanshahi M, Rothwell JC (in preparation). Recovery of function of writing in aphasic hemiplegic patients: evidence from transcranial magnetic stimulation.

Pascual-Leone A, Meador KJ (1998). Is transcranial magnetic stimulation coming of age? Journal of Clinical Neurophysiology 15(4): 285–7.

Powell G (1981). Brain Function Therapy. London: Gower.

Rossini PM, Caltagirone C, Castriota-Scanderbeg A, Cicinelli P, Del Grata C, Demartin M, Pizzela V, Traversa R, Romani GL (1998). Hand motor cortical reorganization in stroke: a study with fMRI, MEG and TCS maps. Neuroreport 9: 2141–6.

Simos P, Breier JI, Zouridakis G, Papanikolaou AC (1998). Assessment of functional cerebral laterality for language using magnetoencephalography. Journal of Clinical Neurophysiology 15(4): 364–72.

Small SL (1994). Connectionist networks and language disorders. Journal of Communication Disorders 27: 305–23.

Stein DG, Glazier MM (1992). An overview of developments in research on recovery from brain injury. Advances in Experimental and Medical Biology 325: 1–22.

Tokimura H, Tokimura Y, Oliviero A, Asakura T, Rothwell JC (1996). Speech-induced changes in corticospinal excitability. Annals of Neurology 40: 628–34.

Topper K, Mottaghy FM, Brugmann M, Noth J, Huber W (1998). Facilitation of picture naming by focal transcranial magnetic stimulation of Wernicke's area. Experimental Brain Research 121: 371–8.

Walker-Batson D, Curtis S, Wolf T, Porch B (1996). Administration of amphetamine accelerates recovery from aphasia. Brain and Language 55(1): 27–9.

Wellier C, Isensee C, Rijintjes M, Huber W, Muller S, Bier D, Dutschka K, Woods RP, Noth J, Diener HC (1995). Recovery from Wernicke's aphasia – a PET study. Annals of Neurology 37: 723–32.

Wepman JM, Jones LV (1961). Language of Modalities for Aphasia. Chicago, IL: Education Industry Service.

Westbury C (1998). Research strategies: psychological and psycholinguistic methods in neurolinguistics. In Stemmer B, Whitaker HA (eds) Handbook of Neurolinguistics. San Diego, CA: Academic Press, pp.84–95.

Whurr R (1982). Towards a linguistic typology in aphasia. In Crystal D (ed.) Linguistic Controversies. London: Edward Arnold, pp.239–55.

Chapter 3
Living with aphasia: a framework for therapy interventions

SALLY BYNG, CAROLE POUND and SUSIE PARR

In the literature on communication impairments there has probably been more written about aphasia than about any other type of impairment. The phenomenon of aphasic language has fascinated, puzzled and inspired researchers and clinicians alike. Yet, as many observers have noted, little substantial attention has been paid in the literature and among researchers to psychosocial issues related to aphasia.

The crucial importance of these issues cannot, however, be denied. Sarno (1993) points out that there has been a skew to the research carried out in the field, and suggests some reasons for this: 'The abrupt and marked alterations aphasia imposes on the person and family – their impact on the life cycle and their continuous influence and evolution – usually for the remainder of the individual's life, have not much appeal to the aphasia research community' (p.322). She suggests that the long-term nature of the aphasic impairment causes it to lack 'the visibility and fascination of the [high-tech] dramas played out in acute care settings' (p.323).

So much research energy has focused on the language impairment that issues about the person have been neglected: '... the quantity, quality and visibility of neurolinguistic study in aphasia have, in some respects, led to a skewed perception of needs and priorities' (Sarno, 1993). Calls for greater attention to these issues have been made with regularity (for example, Tanner and Gerstenberger, 1988; Brumfitt, 1993; Sarno, 1993), but have not resulted in a sustained or substantial research effort. Clinicians are left to deal as best they may with these complex, distressing, interdependent and sometimes apparently impenetrable effects.

What do we mean by 'psychosocial effects' anyway? The way that the term psychosocial is often used in the literature seems to assume some agreed definition of what it comprises. The word itself suggests a combination of the psychological and social effects – a substantial collection of perhaps quite disparate issues. In a recent text on the subject, Lafond et al. (1993) include issues as wide-ranging as psychological effects, employment, leisure, family relationships, effects of bilingualism and ethics. Other writers include effects on functional communication as part of the psychosocial effects.

Psychosocial effects can be summarized into three main categories (see Table 3.1): effects on lifestyle, effects on the person and effects on those in the immediate social context.

Table 3.1. A summary of issues considered under the heading 'psychosocial'

Effects on lifestyle	Effects on person	Effects on others in the immediate social context
employment	psychological effects	identity
education	identity	relationships
leisure	self-esteem and stigma	psychological effects
finances	relationships	role changes
social networks	role changes	
social inclusion		

Of these issues, it would seem that most research has been conducted on depression following stroke, which has been quite well described (for example, Starkstein and Robinson, 1988). The other effects are described (for example, Lafond et al., 1993) but with little explanatory investigation or detailing of appropriate therapeutic intervention.

Not only is there a tendency to cluster all of these issues together under the heading 'psychosocial' but there is also a tendency to imply that similar effects and reactions can be seen in all aphasic people/carers. There seem to be few accounts of why people may react in the way that they do and what prompts these reactions.

In summary, it seems that the term 'psychosocial effects' incorporates everything to do with the impact of aphasia which cannot be included under the heading of language and communication impairment. Herein may lie a problem: this polarization could divorce, at least in the mind of the researcher/reader/clinician, the 'psychosocial' issues from the communication impairment. Yet, in practice, are the two not inextricably linked?

The relationship between communication and language impairment and psychosocial issues

In order to probe this issue further it is helpful to consider the relationship between functional communication (another overused and confusing term) and the psychosocial effects of aphasia. It is here that the interface between the language and communication impairment and 'psychosocial issues' can be most clearly articulated.

The term functional communication has come to have three primary interpretations, clarified by Elman and Bernstein-Ellis (1995). The first is 'getting messages across in a variety of ways ranging from fully-formed grammatical sentences to appropriate gestures, rather than being limited to the use of grammatically correct utterances' (Holland, 1982); that is, enabling someone to convey meaning, regardless of how it is achieved. The second interpretation seems to be task-based: 'which activities are viewed by the aphasic individual as important for their own way of living?' (Smith, 1985). Elman and Bernstein-Ellis (1995) point out that a third definition of functional is creeping in, in order to meet the demands of purchasers or third-party payers – that is, of achieving a set of basic skills. The goal of therapy, within the framework of this definition, becomes to ensure that someone has acquired these basic communicative skills to ensure they have become a 'functional communicator'. Once this has been achieved, therapy is complete, because third-party payers construe that the aims of intervention have been achieved. Furthermore, Simmons (1993) has also drawn attention to the focus by speech and language therapists/pathologists on the *transactional* rather than *interactional* function of communication. Intervention then becomes more strongly related to transfer of information or messages rather than sharing of ideas, thoughts and opinions.

However, as Elman and Bernstein-Ellis point out, the assumption that basic communication skills are adequate to communicate functionally represents a gross oversimplification of what it means to 'function'. This was vividly illustrated by an aphasic man with whom they worked:

> PG was frustrated that a previous facility had terminated therapy because the severity of his aphasia no longer affected 'basic' communicative skills. PG literally shouted to us, 'I am *not* functional!' This retired dentist told us that he could no longer maintain his premorbid role as the joke teller, debater, or group discussant at social or business functions. He pleaded with us to enrol him in our research project so that he could have a chance to regain his personality (pp.115–116).

Elman and Bernstein-Ellis point out that '... although they [aphasic people] are judged functional given a basic skills definition, they are not functional in everyday life.'

To 'function', then, does not mean only to be able to ask for the toilet/a cup of tea/your destination on the bus. To 'function' for PG meant to be a person he could recognize and to play a role that he found acceptable. The 'functional' communication skills PG had acquired did not accord with allowing him to express his *identity*: they restricted his social range, and changed his sense of self and his role in his community. His aphasia had indeed changed his 'function' (what he could do and how he could do it), but it had changed more than that – it had changed how he felt about himself and it had changed for him the world within which he lived.

The aphasia must also have changed the world for those in his immediate social context – PG could no longer be relied on to carry out the roles people expected of him. This must have meant a change or adaptation on the part of other people connected to him too. The effects of the aphasia are therefore not limited to PG or even to his immediate family and friends, but to his community and society more generally. As Goodwin (1995) puts it: 'As an injury aphasia does reside in the skull. However as a form of life, a way of being and acting in the world in concert with others, its proper locus is an endogenous, distributed, multi-party system.' This is undoubtedly true of many other life-transforming illnesses.

There is, therefore, a direct relationship between functional communication and 'psychosocial issues'. Suppose that PG's communication skills did 'improve' to a level where he could express his personality in the way that he wished, to allow him to joke, to be witty, to act as discussant. Would he feel himself to be the way he was before his stroke? And is it realistic to assume that, through intervention by therapists and by himself, his communication skills could be returned to their premorbid style and level? The answer to both those questions is probably no. The aphasia is not going to go away entirely, and even if it did, PG has been through a life-changing experience that is unlikely to leave him being the same person that he was previously. If he is not going to acquire the communication skills that he wants, then he is going to need to find a *modus vivendi* in the context of the communication skills that he does have. The alternative to an inability to find this new way of life is to live striving or waiting to become as he was, a way of life that may become increasingly stressful and dissatisfying.

This clarification is not intended either to be a counsel of despair or to suggest that working on the communication and language impairment is ineffective. Rather it is an acknowledgement that, however much someone's communication skills 'improve', they are never likely (after the acute stage) to return to how they were before the aphasia struck, which in turn means that the person is unlikely to remain 'the same'. People with aphasia have therefore to go through a process of adaptation to these changes.

An equilibrium has therefore to be achieved in intervention between working to enhance communication skills – by working directly on the impairment and on strategies to use skills most effectively – and working on achieving a satisfactory sense of identity, making appropriate and acceptable lifestyle choices. Intervention that focuses on only one side of this equation is not going to be satisfying for the aphasic person or for the therapist; the interrelatedness and interdependency of communication skills and identity is critical. A continuum or reciprocity develops between these issues, as is illustrated in Figure 3.1.

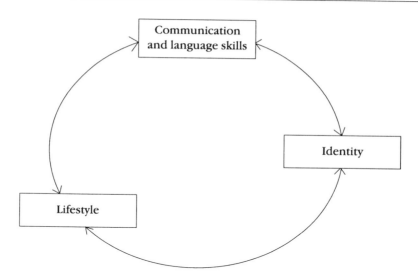

Figure 3.1: The interrelatedness of communication and identity in the process of adaptation to aphasia.

A revised definition of functional communication should perhaps be constructed: being able to communicate competently, through your own communication skills and those of others (see, for example, Kagan, 1998), and feeling comfortable that you are representing who you are.

This definition therefore links inextricably the need for intervention to focus simultaneously on issues to do with identity and issues to do with communication. It also includes those around the person with aphasia as part of the communication chain: the non-aphasic communicator has to have enhanced communication skills, not just the aphasic person, to allow the aphasic person to communicate effectively, as has been so clearly demonstrated by Lyon (Lyon, 1997, 1998; Lyon et al., 1997), Kagan and Gailey (1993) and Simmons-Mackie and Damico (1997). Aphasia becomes a systemic issue, insoluble by the aphasic person alone, requiring change not only on the part of the aphasic person, but also on the part of those in the person's immediate social context, the community and in society in general – a tall order, but not unachievable.

The systemic effects of aphasia

Much of the conceptualization of aphasia has been at the level of the individual: for example, Sarno (1993: 323) suggests that 'Aphasia can be perceived as a disorder of communication leading to a disorder of person.' The statement conveys that the problems are focused on the individual and the aphasia is construed as a disorder – something that is wrong. This puts the definition in a frame of reference belonging to a medical model of disability, which underpins the definitions of disability that have been used by the World Health Organization. They focus on the *inabilities* of the impaired individual, and on the assumed goal of cure or improvement, while the disability is seen to stem directly from the impairment, and is itself the focus for treatment or cure.

A more radical definition of disability (and one which is challenging to professional groups concerned with rehabilitation) has been developed by members of the disability movement in the United Kingdom. According to this definition, disability arises not from the impaired individual's inability to perform normal activities, but from the barriers and restrictions imposed by society on the impaired person.

Disability therefore becomes 'the loss or limitation of opportunities that prevents people who have impairments from taking part in the normal life of the community on an equal level with others due to physical and social barriers' (Finkelstein and French, 1993: 28). Defined in this way, disability becomes something that can be mitigated not by treatment or cure, but by recognition and removal of the barriers. It places the individual at the heart of communities who take responsibility for their role in mitigating the impact of the disability. Although this account of disability has some limitations, it is provocative in forcing us to think about whether there may not be externally imposed barriers exacerbating the social exclusion experienced by people with aphasia.

The impact of this construction of disability, alongside the already acknowledged need to modify the communication environment to enable the aphasic person to communicate competently, leads us to set a wider perspective on the targets for intervention for someone with aphasia. It is no longer sufficient to confine our intervention to one-to-one therapy with the aphasic person, since the aphasia is not just the problem of the individual and its effects can be exacerbated by society.

Writers from within the disability movement have also drawn attention to the perspective from which much writing about disability stems. Oliver (1996) provocatively remarks that rehabilitation traditionally 'denies the subjective experience of disablement' and suggests that the personal story has political potential. All too often, research into disability reflects the 'outsider perspective' or the professional view of the issue, not that of the person experiencing the disability or the 'insider' perspective (Conrad, 1990). This has been all too true within the aphasia literature on psychosocial issues.

Insider and outsider perspectives on psychosocial issues: aphasia and identity

In a now well-known paper on what is described as the grief response following aphasia, Tanner and Gerstenberger (1988: 79) suggest that 'There are three dimensions of loss experienced by patients with neuropathologies of speech and language: person, self and object.'

There is an underlying assumption to this statement that these three losses are common to all people with aphasia. This reflects much of the literature on psychosocial issues: it is written from the perspective of the professional, the researcher who is usually an outsider in relation to the condition. Descriptions of, and explanations for, psychosocial issues are not often made by people with aphasia – that is by people who can give insider accounts.

In a qualitative study we carried out (Parr, Byng and Gilpin, 1997), during which the long-term experience of aphasic people was explored in depth through their own words, a more complex picture emerged of the wide variety of factors that shape and influence what happens to them and how they react to becoming aphasic:

> Progressing through the event of acute illness, treatment and recovery, the aphasic person will find a number of different accounts and identities useful. Coping in this sense, is a messy and untidy business. There are no neat stages through which the aphasic person progresses in an orderly and predictable manner (p.114).

This raises issues about the nature of identities, personal, social and collective, and how these new identities are accommodated – issues which have received attention in the disability literature (for example, Peters (1996) and Corker (1996)). In aphasia there is an added factor – the aphasic person is, of course, engaged in this process of adaptation or accommodation using the medium which is itself impaired (Brumfitt, 1993). Hughes and Paterson (1997) describe the centrality of language to the process of making sense of an impairment: 'Language and metaphor are vehicles for making sense of bodily sensations and actions. In order to turn sensation into sense or meaning language is necessary. Without language, one cannot make sense of an impairment' (p.332). Brumfitt (1993) further elaborates this dilemma: 'What is even less clear is whether aphasics can gain sufficient sense from construing and under-standing their impairment to allow them to develop a strong sense of identity' (p.573).

What is the relationship between understanding the nature of the impairment and development of new identities? In the course of the qualitative interviewing that we undertook we asked people to describe the difficulty they had talking. What emerged was a confusing picture for anyone trying to create a definition of aphasia on the basis of what was said. People were able to describe vividly and sometimes with interesting use of imagery what it felt like emotionally to have their communication difficulties, for example 'a rose tightly shut and a bit wilting' (Rose) or 'I had a hole in my head and I could see the words tumbling down there' (Les). However, when it came to describing what was wrong or where the problem lay, then much more difficulty was experienced.

People who had lived with the experience of aphasia for more than 5 years did not always know what had caused their communication problems: some interpreted it as a form of laryngitis, whereas the majority knew it was something related to the brain but were no more clear than that. Strikingly few people could describe their difficulties in any detail. There is a sense that even the symptoms are hard for people to capture for themselves. This contrasts perhaps with accounts of experiences of physical and other sensory disabilities that offer lengthy descriptions of how they are perceived and experienced (for example, Sacks, 1984, Bauby, 1997). Descriptions of the symptoms of aphasia rarely got beyond describing the feeling that although someone knows what they want to say, they cannot find the word. This suggests that aphasia is a particularly difficult impairment to grasp, even for those who live with it. This has implications for the creation of not only personal and social identities but also collective identities: how do people with aphasia construe other people with aphasia?

Brumfitt (1993) describes the aphasic person as having a 'fundamental need to develop an alternative and new sense of self if he or she is to adapt to forced changes' (p.572). Identity seems, then, to be inextricably linked to functional outcome. Furthermore, it seems that both understanding the nature of the impairment and having the underpinning skills to promote good communication may be critical to the process of adaptation. Any process of learning to live with aphasia is going to require an integration of interventions designed to meet this range of needs: an uneven focus on one issue only could mean the omission of a critical link in the process of recapturing life after aphasia.

Implications for therapy intervention

This close interrelationship of all the factors related to how someone finds a way of living with their aphasia calls for a model of provision of intervention by therapy services which represents an integrated framework. In order to provide a context for the framework we need to be clear about what the ultimate outcome of intervention represents. We propose a definition that encompasses the aim of all intervention in aphasia, which is to promote, however indirectly, healthy living with aphasia. 'Healthy' is interpreted broadly here to include both mental and physical health. A framework for therapy intervention needs to reflect both the necessarily systemic targets for therapy and the integration of therapies focusing on all aspects of the impact of aphasia, what might be called 'impact-led intervention' (Rucker, 1998). Figure 3.2 provides a schematic representation of a framework for intervention.

In the remainder of this chapter we will go on to articulate this framework, providing examples of therapy interventions related to the major goals. Finally, we will exemplify the operation of the framework through two short case descriptions.

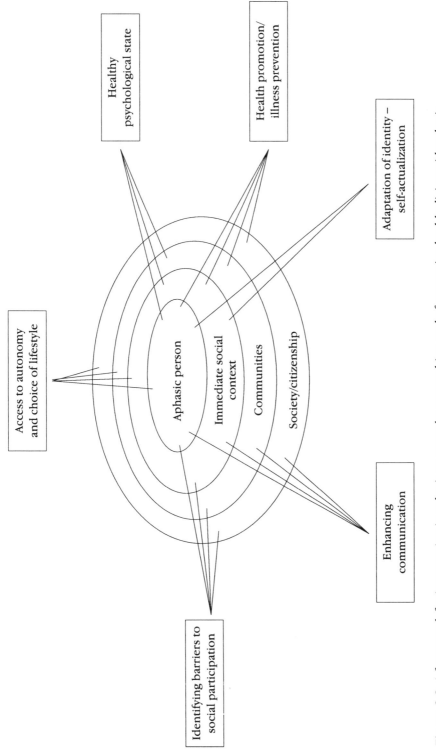

Figure 3.2: A framework for intervention in aphasia to meet the overarching goal of promoting healthy living with aphasia.

The framework represents the need for intervention to address the systemic nature of the effects of aphasia. The person with aphasia is at the centre of the framework, surrounded not only by those in the immediate environment, but also by communities, for example, neighbourhood, family, work, education, leisure interests, religious communities and so on, and by society more generally.

Means of addressing each of the major goals can be exemplified. For some of them the literature is rich with illustrations, for example, the impairment-based therapies, whereas others have been barely considered in formal descriptions of therapy, for example, interventions focusing on identity and self-actualization. Table 3.2 sets out some examples of the type of therapy programmes that might be undertaken to address each of the major goals. Sometimes one major goal can, itself, represent a means of addressing another goal. For example, enhancing communication can be a major goal or a means of addressing health promotion or illness prevention. Alternatively, one therapy programme can address two different goals simultaneously. What comes across clearly from this table is the interdependency of one goal on another; the process of learning to live well with aphasia cannot be achieved without an integrated and rounded set of interventions being provided.

Note that the words psychosocial or functional do not appear in this framework. Rather, it serves to illustrate the necessary interrelatedness and interdependency of interventions. It sets a context for each individual type of intervention, which helps to clarify the goals of individual therapies. For example, working to enhance the communication impairment is woven into a number of different overall goals. This crystallizes the purpose of the intervention, thus serving to clarify in the mind of the therapist, as well as of the aphasic person, the direction that the therapy is taking and its contribution to promoting healthy living with aphasia, however small or indirect. This may make a difference to the way in which the therapy is delivered.

In the remainder of this section we will illustrate what some of the therapy approaches/programmes outlined in Table 3.2 entail. Some are familiar and have a rich set of exemplars in the literature; others less so.

Intervention goals and therapy programmes

Enhancing communication

This goal represents that which perhaps has been most familiar to therapists. The aim of this goal could perhaps be stated as 'achieving maximum potential for communication by enhancing both the communication skills of the aphasic person and the skills of those with whom they communicate'. There is an implicit understanding that communication here represents both interaction and transaction (Simmons, 1993); that is that therapy needs not just to enable the aphasic person to

Table 3.2: Interventions designed to address the major goals of intervention in aphasia

Goals of intervention	Examples of intervention programmes (not an exclusive or exhaustive list) e.g.			
	Individual	Immediate social context	Communities	Society/citizenship
Enhancing communication	• impairment-based therapies • communication strategies	• enhancing communication skills of care-givers	• conversation partners	• educational packages
Adaptation of identity	• self-advocacy • personal portfolios • counselling • self-help groups	• enhancing communication • counselling • care-givers' groups		
Access to autonomy and choice of lifestyle	• access to information • personal portfolios • enhancing communication • self-advocacy	• enhancing communication • access to information	• educational packages for employers, leisure and education service providers, etc.	• information • educational packages for policy makers, social and healthcare service providers
Identifying barriers to social participation	• provision of accessible information • self-advocacy	• enhancing communication	• advocacy	• environmental modifications • educational and training packages
Health promotion/ illness prevention	• stress management • self-assertiveness • enhancing communication	• care-givers' groups	• information and educational packages and training for service providers	• information and educational packages for and training
Healthy psychological state	• counselling • pharmacological interventions • self-advocacy • psychotherapy	• pharmacological interventions • psychotherapy • family therapy • counselling	• access to information • support for differential diagnosis	

transmit information but also to engage in the exchange of ideas, thoughts and opinions which represent a reflection of who they are. In this way enhancing communication also serves to facilitate expression of identity. Davidson, Worrall and Hickson (1998) have demonstrated that people with aphasia spend much less time telling stories in everyday communication than non-aphasic people. Stories represent an important means of expressing identity, so this striking difference suggests the importance of facilitating a wide range of types of communication.

A variety of means of achieving enhanced communication can be employed and the following categories represent some of the programmes that might be used:

(i) Impairment-based therapies

The impairment itself may be directly addressed. This is where the bulk of the research in aphasia has been carried out. Addressing the impairment directly includes therapies that aim to change or modify aspects of the impaired language (for example, Helm-Estabrooks and Ramsberger, 1986; Jones, 1986; Marshall, Pring and Chiat, 1993; Thompson, Shapiro and Roberts, 1993; and Lesser and Algar, 1995). The theoretical approach underlying these therapies may vary from, for example, a stimulation approach through to a localizationist approach or to a cognitive neuropsychological approach. What they have in common is that they are trying to change the language and communication difficulties themselves, by some clearly specified means.

(ii) Communication strategies

The development of strategies to find a way around the language impairments, rather than tackling them head on, has been well defined by aphasiologists over the past two decades (for example, Aten, Caligiuri and Holland, 1982; McCrae Cochrane and Milton, 1984; Davis and Wilcox, 1985; Holland, 1991; Lesser and Algar, 1995). The impetus for this work was both to circumvent the language impairment and to supplement the means of communication to be used by the aphasic person. It stemmed from the observation that aphasic people are better communicators than talkers and often have at their disposal a number of different means and modalities of communication that they can employ. These strategies aim to make the most of all these means.

(iii) Conversation partners (Kagan and Gailey, 1993; Lyon et al., 1997; Kagan, 1998)

This represents a newer concept and focuses on providing individuals with opportunities for genuine adult conversation and interaction by emphasizing less the use of independent communication strategies by the aphasic partner in a conversation, and more what the conversational dyad achieves *interdependently* (Kagan, 1998). The intervention still has the aim of enhancing the experience of communication, but this time the focus is not on changing the impairment in some way but on changing the 'environment' of the communication. The onus on changing communication skills is not all on the person with aphasia, but also on the persons with whom they are communicating to adapt and modify their style of communication to include and support the aphasic person, revealing their communicative competence (Kagan, 1995). Kagan makes a cogent case for the implications of this type of intervention also enhancing identity and psychological state by reducing social isolation. In this way the critical interdependence and interrelatedness of interventions is yet again underlined.

(iv) Enhancing the communication skills of care-givers and others in the immediate social environment

Care-givers are not necessarily the communication partners referred to by Kagan and others above. Often the approaches aimed at training conversation partners are specifically introducing different types of partner, allowing opportunities for communication outside the usual home or residential environment. However, the principle underlying the need for spouses, partners, residential care staff, family members and friends to change their communication skills to accommodate the aphasic person remains the same: the communicative competence of the aphasic person cannot be revealed without the non-aphasic partner supporting their attempts to communicate. Sacchett and colleagues (1999) demonstrated that, for alternative forms of communication to be of use, the most immediate communication partners have also to learn interpretation skills and to modify their own output. Could it be that in some cases it may be more efficient to use the therapy resource to modify the communication skills of those around the aphasic person than to change the aphasic person's communication? This might be a fruitful avenue for cost-benefit analysis.

These four examples of means of enhancing communication serve as illustrations of interventions that aim to address more or less directly the communication difficulties caused by the aphasia. There are many examples of each kind and other categories that have not been included: the ideas here serve merely as examples of the kinds of interventions commonly used to address the aim of enhancing communication.

Adaptation of identity

The overall goal of establishing an identity as a person with aphasia has not been explicitly expressed until relatively recently (for example, Brumfitt, 1993), yet the changes experienced are clearly profound (Parr, Byng and Gilpin, 1997). The need expressed by Elman and

Bernstein-Ellis' subject PC (Elman and Bernstein-Ellis, 1995) referred to earlier is heartfelt. Clearly, people need considerable support and sometimes specific intervention in establishing this revision to their identity and personal biography (Kleinman, 1988). This may include, at a personal level, the following issues:

- finding a way to maintain a former sense of self and forge a new identity which accommodates the aphasia, incorporating changes to a personal biography;
- acknowledging the losses and struggles encountered and identifying gains;
- accessing new ideas, interests, roles and relationships;
- living with aphasia without persistently damaging self-esteem by apologizing for it (Parr et al., 1997);
- identifying the source of the problem as often outside the individual rather than always within.
  There may also be some issues to do with creating a group identity:
- identifying themes common to the personal struggles of the self and also others with aphasia;
- discussing and exploring awareness, ignorance and attitudes in society;
- collective campaigning against discrimination and poor public awareness;
- sharing experience and developing trusting relationships to counter isolation and exclusion.

Table 3.2 identifies some specific interventions through which these issues may be explored:

(i) Self-advocacy

Self-advocacy involves three main features – enhancing self-esteem, developing skills and knowledge, and personal and collective empowerment. In order to achieve this empowerment Pound (1998) suggests that people who are learning to be self-advocates need to develop the following:

- a strong sense of self and a positive self-image;
- an awareness of strengths and skills rather than a focus on impairments;
- an awareness and critical consciousness of the current social and political situation;
- a sense of the importance of participation in community; and
- an involvement in the process as collaborators rather than service recipients.

Pound (1998) and Penman (1998) describe two linked experimental self-advocacy groups run in parallel. Part of the process of the groups' attempts to become self-advocates involved the development of personal portfolios. These acted as extended curriculum vitae, which linked the past, future and current selves of the participants. These groups were evaluated by qualitative means, which demonstrated both the enthusiasm for the work and the groups' perceptions that they had achieved the goals that they had set themselves. Participants felt that they had moved on personally as a result of the group in a way that they had not experienced through other group therapies.

(ii) Care-givers' groups and self-help groups

Groups can provide a powerful medium for addressing many complex issues that may be experienced by both people with aphasia and care-givers (Holland and Beeson, 1999) and represent a significant thera-peutic tool. They offer an exciting and dynamic medium through which many of the issues related to living with aphasia can be addressed most effectively.

Aphasic people are not the only ones whose identities have changed as a result of the aphasia. Clearly, the lives of those around the aphasic person have changed so that their identities have changed also (Carnwath and Johnson, 1987; Anderson, 1992). A participant in a group for care-givers (Pound and Parr, in preparation) described how she had changed; 'It's frightening because I have no future. I'm an orderly person and suddenly it's changing and it's quite distressing. I can't tidy up because everything is going to change.'

Groups run for carers can provide psychological support (Rice, Paull and Muller, 1987) and more specifically can help people to gain a sense of identity (Pound and Parr, in preparation). This identity may challenge the conventional view of the spouse as 'carer'.

Self-help groups are gaining in impetus as a means of finding a creative way for aphasic people to work together to find new ways of establishing their identity. 'Self help is about personal responsibility and interdependence... Its ethos is empowering and enabling rather than protective, prescriptive and philanthropic' (The Joseph Rowntree Foundation, 1995). Therapists may play a role in facilitating the creation of groups and act as a resource in sustaining them.

(iii) Enhancing communication

This would seem to be a logical step in facilitating adaptation to identity – the more access to satisfying communication, the more possibilities there may be to develop a new or changed identity. However, a note of caution may be worth sounding here: too much emphasis on impaired language can, for someone who is striving to adapt to a new identity, just reinforce the negative aspects of what they can no longer do. Thus, work on the language impairment may have to be negotiated delicately and sensitively with someone who is acquiring a new, positive sense of self.

(iv) Counselling

Counselling has been part of the therapeutic armoury for some time, and can be used with both aphasic people and care-givers in the pursuit of support for adaptation to new identities. One aphasic recipient of counselling described the sometimes intangible benefits of counselling: 'I didn't put perfume on, whereas I do put perfume on when I go out ... I'd just have a quick wash ... whereas now I have a shower. I wouldn't even comb my hair. You know ... was sloppy' (Ireland and Wootton, 1996: 589).

Access to autonomy and choice of lifestyle

Determining for yourself what you want to do with your life, having some control over that process and ending up doing something that you choose is all too often not a familiar experience or even an option for people with aphasia. Although there may be many different barriers to having this control, frequently it is the aphasia that gets in the way: 'I'm better off than I've ever been. But I'm not better off because I haven't got a life' (Parr et al., 1997: 43).

People with aphasia may need a lot of support in determining both what the range of choices is for them and how they might realize those choices. Inevitably there will be barriers – some caused directly by the aphasia and others at a societal level. Inevitably also, the aphasic persons will have to promote their own cause, hence the need for self-advocacy as one of the intervention options to facilitate teasing out what might be realistic lifestyle opportunities and a means of achieving them.

Access to information about potential opportunities, such as availability of adult education classes, leisure pursuits and welfare benefits to assist in affording these opportunities can be hugely difficult for people with aphasia. Thus, facilitating access to information and thereby to participation in decision making becomes an important area for intervention: 'The thing is, I don't know what I'm entitled to. If you don't know where to start you never get nowhere. I don't know. And it's not just a matter of scared' (Parr et al., 1997: 92). *The Aphasia Handbook* (Parr et al., 1999), an information resource written in a style accessible to people with aphasia, will provide some assistance to aphasic people in finding their way through the maze which is the access route to both services and benefits.

Providers of the kinds of leisure and educational opportunities that people may be seeking, or potential employers, may need support in knowing how to make their services accessible, to facilitate and support the language environment, to take into account the specific needs of people with aphasia and to understand the multiple manifestations of aphasia, for example. So few people return to work after becoming aphasic. How much this is due to the inflexibility of the workplace or ignorance on the part of employers about how to support an aphasic employee, rather than the severity of the aphasia, is hard to estimate. What is clear from individual examples is that, for a number of people with aphasia, adequate support, modification of the environment and identification of sources of difficulty can facilitate either the resumption of previous employment or access to new, alternative forms of employment.

Identifying barriers to social participation

Parr et al. (1997) begin to detail some of the barriers experienced by people with aphasia that prevent access to social participation and lead to social isolation and exclusion. These barriers were identified by aphasic people as including:

* environmental barriers, including noise, the language environment, or time
* structural barriers, including inappropriate, inadequate or inaccessible services, systems or resources
* attitudinal barriers, which include the stigma attached to being unable to communicate, the fear evidenced by people about talking with someone who has difficulty communicating
* informational barriers, which we have described above – where information is again either inaccessible because it is not made available in a form which people can understand or when aphasic people cannot locate the information.

In order to be addressed, these issues require the development of educational and information packages for use by people with aphasia and also for people who provide health and social care services, and adult education and leisure service providers. They require a sustained programme of raising public awareness, which can be achieved through these educational means and through advocacy and self-advocacy. A better understanding of the environmental barriers experienced by aphasic people might facilitate more active addressing of these barriers. For example, understanding how the language environment could be modified in the workplace or at community meetings might facilitate the involvement of aphasic people. This might involve writing minutes of meetings in an aphasia-friendly style, modifying the timing, duration and organization of meetings to permit people with aphasia to participate without becoming lost in the speed and density of the language used, and setting clear ground-rules for participation to take into account specific communication needs.

With the increasing emphasis at a policy level on shared involvement in decision making by 'patients' with health and social care providers, the imperative to find ways of ensuring methods to promote inclusivity· is becoming political as well as ideological. This involvement requires that all parties to the decision making have access to appropriate information and materials with which to inform that decision making. For people with aphasia this means information not only about the range of potential options, but also information about how to communicate them, for all parties to the decision making. Again, this highlights the need for improved awareness of how to modify communication by health and social care providers and others.

Health promotion/illness prevention

The work of therapists is being construed increasingly in terms of promoting good health and preventing secondary effects of illness (Levenson and Farrell, 1998). One role in intervention with aphasia might relate to preparing people for the situations that they might find difficult. This can be achieved through groups run to promote self-assertiveness or management of stress. These groups can anticipate events that might happen in stressful situations. Identifying these situations, exploring what makes them stressful, examining the components and then practising both strategies to minimize stress and to deal with it when it happens, can provide preventative strategies for people to implement. In this way aphasic people can learn explicitly how to take responsibility for aspects of their mental health.

Care-givers' groups can perform the same function with partners. Identifying what makes communication difficult, and what behaviours are particularly difficult to deal with, a partner can identify preventative or avoiding strategies. These may be communication-related, hence the inclusion of enhancing communication, on all sides, as a means of preventing illness, mental or ultimately physical.

Healthy psychological state

Probably more has been written about intervention for the aphasic person's psychological state than for any other aspect of the psychosocial effects of aphasia, so we will refer to it only briefly here. There are a range of therapy interventions that may be appropriate, from counselling through to full-scale psychotherapy (Ireland, 1995). Clinical depression does appear to be one of the major sequelae of stroke that is often underestimated and neglected (Starkstein and Robinson, 1988). Endogenous and reactive depressions are not unusual and may be treated pharmacologically.

The form that the depression takes may differ in the acute and chronic stages post-stroke. The impact of the stroke and the aphasia may also create depression for those in the immediate social context, and may also require intervention. Family therapies have been proposed and evaluated by Wahrborg and Borenstein (1989) and Nichols, Varchevker and Pring (1996).

There may often be a role for the speech and language therapist either in ensuring that pharmaceutical information is understood by someone with aphasia or that other professionals provide this in an accessible form. There is also a need to support differential diagnosis in cases where the psychological state of the aphasic person is difficult to determine because of the aphasia.

Clinical reality

Although this framework provides a basis for conceptualizing intervention, the exemplars of its implementation look too neat and tidy to reflect clinical reality. In practice, how does this work? Clinicians know all too well the multiplicity of factors that have to be taken into account in putting together and agreeing any package of therapy: resource issues, the personality of the aphasic person or therapist, their priorities, their health beliefs, the complexities of their immediate social environment, family dynamics and crises, ongoing life events and financial uncertainty. All of these issues impact on the formulation of the goals of intervention and the treatment array (Elman, 1998) which can be made available. They form an 'overlay' or context, which shapes the course of the intervention, sometimes in conflict with the goals the therapist or the aphasic person would like to pursue.

People experience aphasia in the context of the course of life events, changes, crises and celebrations that all of us experience. This means that the needs of people with aphasia can change dramatically, even if their aphasia does not. The death of a care-giver can mean a radical change in lifestyle, which might bring with it new demands on communication skills, even years after the onset of aphasia. Some means of providing short-term intervention or support in such cases should be considered. All too often, intervention services are focused at the onset of aphasia and are not sufficiently flexible to address ongoing issues. Aphasia is an event that becomes a process. This means that therapy intervention needs to be flexible and dynamic, involving periodic stock-taking and revision of goals and directions, incorporating the range of levels of working identified here.

To illustrate the clinical reality of implementing this framework of interventions the following section will illustrate two 'packages' of intervention for two clients who have attended the aphasia centre at City University. These two vignettes convey the need in therapy to address the interrelatedness and interdependency of the goals of intervention, and changes in goals over time, to achieve the overall aim of living healthily with aphasia.

Betty

Betty was 64 years old when she had a large left-hemisphere stroke leaving her with severe receptive and expressive aphasia and a dense right hemiplegia. One year prior to her stroke she had retired from a long career as a shop assistant. About 18 months after her stroke, her husband of more than 40 years died and after a short period living with her daughter and her family, Betty moved into sheltered accommodation. Prior to her stroke she was reported to have been sociable and outgoing, enjoying shopping, gardening, music and singing.

Prior to beginning therapy at the aphasia centre, Betty had received an 8-month period of hospital inpatient and outpatient therapy and a period of outpatient neurorehabilitation following her move to sheltered accommodation. Betty had been discharged from both services with reports of limited progress in therapy, continuing global aphasia and marked anxiety in all communicative situations.

When Betty began attending the centre for a package of individual communication therapy and counselling she had been aphasic for more than 2 years. On admission to the centre she required constant one-to-one supervision when walking, waiting and accessing refreshments and was emotionally labile throughout sessions. Speech was unintelligible and consisted of recurrent neologistic utterances and, although she demonstrated some ability to write single words, spontaneous attempts to communicate through writing consisted of lists of semantically and/or orthographically related words and part-words which bore no apparent relationship to the topic in hand.

Initially, individual therapy with Betty had a strong focus on enhancing communication with an impairment focus, using a combination of semantic-based choices and written word copying to develop Betty's ability to use writing communicatively. Betty remained extremely labile in sessions, emotional responses being repeatedly prompted by any reference to previous life experiences, hobbies, and family events relating to her deceased husband, Eric.

Soon after coming to the centre, however, Betty began sessions with the stroke counsellor, Harry, to address the urgent issues related to her psychological state. At this time Betty had very limited means of self-expression and seemed to spend most of her time with Harry either sobbing or pointing repeatedly and quizzically to her mouth. As single-word written output developed and Harry experimented with use of painting, drawing and singing, Betty seemed more able to restrict her tearful episodes within language therapy sessions, and family and therapists observed Betty taking a more confident, independent role in communicative interactions and increased spontaneous use of single written words to express ideas. One year into her therapy at the centre Betty was able to interact independently with new students, centre staff and taxi drivers and became distressed only when faced with the unexpected or transport difficulties.

Contact with Betty's family during this time was largely limited to telephone contact due to work and other pressures, but a long-standing friend came to a carers' support group where issues of coping with guilt, frustration and depression were common topics of discussion, along with video tips for conversation partner training.

As Betty's communicative ability (using writing and total communication techniques) and confidence continued to develop, therapy began to focus on developing a 'conversation' folder to support Betty in communicating non-verbally with friends and family and to represent her life and identity. Betty was encouraged to take a full and active role in selecting and organizing pictorial material. Throughout this period Betty continued to attend weekly counselling sessions which focused on non-verbal discussion and demonstration of her feelings about her loss of language and the loss of her husband.

Sadly, towards the end of her second year in therapy, Betty suffered a series of seizures and falls which adversely affected her confidence in travelling alone to the centre. There was also evidence of a decline in cognitive and communicative skills at this time. Prior to a further period of ill-health and hospitalization, a volunteer was trained in supported conversation techniques (Kagan, 1998) in order to visit Betty at home for weekly conversations based around the interests and life events she had depicted in her conversation folder.

Goals of intervention with Betty focused, simultaneously and in sequence, on enhancing communication (both hers and that of her friends and family), on her psychological state, on adaptation to her new identity as a widow and as a person with a severe communication impairment and on providing new opportunities for self-expression and participation. Her friends and family were also supported in coping with her communication and psychological needs, providing some support to contain the stress and anxiety they were experiencing. Removing any one of this complex and interacting range of interventions would have diminished the effectiveness of the whole.

Valerie

Valerie was 42 years old and had just completed a Masters degree in politics when she had a subarachnoid haemorrhage and neurosurgical interventions to clip three aneurysms. At the time of her haemorrhage she was single and working more than full-time as a researcher for a trade union. Her passions were walking, reading and socializing with a wide network of work-related colleagues. She was about to embark on a PhD.

Subsequent to her illness and periods of intensive rehabilitation at specialist neurological hospitals, neurorehabilitation units and through a community therapy team, she remained moderately aphasic and had persisting mobility difficulties, although she could walk independently with a stick.

At one year post-stroke she began attending the aphasia centre at City University 2 days a week for an integrated package of individual and group therapies. Having recently spent 3 months as an inpatient at a neurorehabilitation unit, Valerie came to the centre asking for more therapy to improve her talking and reading and an almost unquenchable thirst for impairment-based worksheets which might address these goals. Her initial contacts with other group members were cordial but slightly detached and her anger and withdrawal were frequently apparent when the topic of conversation addressed issues around living with aphasia. On other occasions and as time progressed, her rage about the ignorant and patronising attitudes of people towards individuals with disabilities and her sadness and fear about an uncertain future formed passionate inputs to group discussions.

Valerie participated in a range of themed groups aimed at exploring her own and others' internal and external barriers to a more comfortable co-existence with aphasia and disability. These included:

- a group project to develop an accessible, aphasia-friendly leaflet about the centre – this involved not only discussion about the nature and impact of aphasia but much thought and problem-solving regarding how to represent the bizarreness of aphasia in a concrete, digestible way;
- an assertiveness and aphasia group – which interestingly contrasted Valerie's outwardly assertive style with her constant apologies for her speech;
- a group which explored ways and means of training conversation partners or people with aphasia – which enabled her to give vent to her feelings about the friends and acquaintances who still showed no awareness of her needs in social interactions;
- a poetry and aphasia group which looked at ways of re-experiencing literature and accessing her former love of poetry;
- a portfolio group in which she compiled a life history bringing together her family and geographical roots, her high-achieving worklife, and, ultimately, the most difficult subject of all, her interpretation of her illness, path of recovery and aspirations for the future.

Alongside these programmes she spent individual sessions which built on earlier impairment-based goals and began moving new skills and strategies into a more work-oriented arena. These therapies included:

- semantic-based verb therapy
- developing reading strategies
- searching written information for selected information

- summarizing written information from newspapers about her key research areas
- developing competence and confidence in using email and the internet, a technological revolution that had coincided with her time away from work and a skill which would enable Valerie to meet her long-term goal of working from home at her own pace.

In addition to these sessions, towards the end of her therapy at the centre, Valerie began weekly counselling with the specialist stroke counsellor, a service that she had for many months felt unable to take up as she felt 'too sad'. Here, she further reflected on changes and challenges to her ability to integrate her former identity and lifestyle with the new person she was struggling to be since her life-changing haemorrhage.

After 18 months at the centre Valerie expressed a desire to finish therapy. Although the prospect of a part-time return to work had not yet been implemented, Valerie was looking forward, although not without some trepidation, to spending time at home on her computer and experimenting with a new way of working.

Valerie's journey through therapy again illustrates the interwoven goals of intervention. She needed to continue to work on her impairment and, indeed, seemed to resist any other focus. But by working in an environment where a wider range of opportunities for intervention were available, she became able to take them up and use them at the point at which she could deal with them emotionally. Had she not had the opportunity to consider overtly issues to do with negotiating barriers to social exclusion, re-establishing her identity and identifying realistically lifestyle choices, alongside work on enhancing communication (again both hers and that of her social network), what would the outcomes have been? Could she have done all the necessary 'inside work' (Parr et al., 1997) and identified barriers on her own, while therapy focused on her language?

Continuing complexities

Although we believe that the framework offered here clarifies a range of legitimate goals for intervention in aphasia, many complexities remain. For example, what means of assessing or investigating need should underpin these approaches? How can the effectiveness of the full range of these forms of intervention be evaluated? It is unlikely that conventional forms of speech and language therapy assessment and evaluation methods will be appropriate to meet the requirements of all these forms of intervention. Does this range of intervention imply the need for different kinds of therapeutic skills and do speech and language therapists necessarily have them?

Perhaps this question poses another – who should provide the interventions outlined here? Are they necessarily best addressed by a speech and language therapist, or should they involve other health and social care professionals, either independently or working in collaboration with speech and language therapists? Sarno (1993) suggests that 'The primary goal of rehabilitation is to restore the person's role as a communicator, regardless of whether certain symptoms have been eradicated or particular linguistic skills have improved.' Does this mean that issues to do with social role and identity, for example, are not appropriate goals of rehabilitation, or at least rehabilitation provided by speech and language therapists? Or does 'role as communicator' subsume the notion of social roles as well?

The relative timing of these interventions also bears further consideration. Lyon (1998) suggests that 'we need to shift and look beyond clinical repair from the beginning of therapy, and allot time and support to managing the social dilemmas of people coping with aphasia in real life.' Traditionally, 'psychosocial' considerations have followed a preliminary focus on addressing the impairment. What would the impact be of dealing more overtly with identity and lifestyle issues earlier, as soon as someone has returned home after a period of hospitalization? It is clear that to meet the needs of a person adapting to life with aphasia, an ongoing process of sensitive negotiation and regular renegotiation about directions in intervention is critical.

As we pointed out at the start of this chapter, the history of aphasia therapy could be characterized as one of regular polarizations – between impairment and disability, clinician and researcher, quantitative and qualitative approaches, functional and impairment-based therapies, or different theoretical accounts of the language impairment, for example. Listening to the experiences of aphasic people, the lack of creativity inherent in these polarizations is evident. Aphasic people are asking us, directly and indirectly, to provide interventions that address both their communication impairments and the effects of those impairments on their lives. Sometimes that intervention will involve working directly with aphasic people, sometimes with care-givers or health and social care professionals, sometimes as political and social campaigners and advocates, sometimes as researchers and commentators. We cannot all play all of these roles, but we need to ensure that they are all represented somewhere in the therapy and support system. An intervention provider or researcher who focuses only on one of these aspects is missing out on components of the process of recovery and adaptation which are critical for somebody, at some stage.

It would be unfortunate if the new focus of 'disability' therapy were to create a further polarization. What we have tried to illustrate here is that all therapy interventions are interdependent and work on many different levels simultaneously. Working on the language impairment to enhance communication can also be construed as addressing issues to do with disability. For example, improving auditory input analysis skills might not only improve ability to hear minimal pair contrasts and thereby increase access to the language system as a whole, but also facilitate greater social participation by reducing the confusion and 'noise' experienced through hearing unrecognizable language. It becomes not just an impairment-level intervention but also a means of increasing involvement in shared decision making, for example. Similarly, a self-advocacy group through which individuals become more clear and confident about their identity and choice of lifestyle as people with aphasia, can enable them to identify a specific aspect of the language impairment as a focus for intervention to meet a particular access need. Rather than pigeonholing approaches as either impairment-based or functional- or disability-focused (for example), we should be aiming to clarify what role or roles, in the bigger picture of overall goals of intervention, a specific intervention might play.

These issues bear considerable further elaboration, but what is becoming increasingly clear from much current writing is that the role of the speech and language therapist, who is intervening in the process of recovery from aphasia, is changing and extending, pushed not only by our paymasters but also, and perhaps more importantly, by people with aphasia. We have no choice but to listen to them and act accordingly.

References

Anderson R (1992) The Aftermath of Stroke. Cambridge: Cambridge University Press.

Aten J, Caligiuri MP, Holland A (1982). The efficacy of functional communication therapy for chronic aphasic patients. Journal of Speech and Hearing Disorders 47: 93–6.

Bauby J-D (1997) The Diving Bell and the Butterfly. London: Fourth Estate.

Brumfitt S (1993). Losing your sense of self: What aphasia can do. Clinical Forum in Aphasiology 7(6): 569–91.

Carnwath CM, Johnson DAW (1987). Psychiatric morbidity among spouses of patients with stroke. British Medical Journal 294: 409–11.

Conrad P (1990). Qualitative research on chronic illness: a commentary on method and conceptual development. Social Science of Medicine 30(11): 1257–63.

Corker M (1996). Deaf Transitions: Images and Origins of Deaf Families, Deaf Communities and Deaf Identities. London: Jessica Kingsley.

Davidson B, Worrall L, Hickson L (1998). Observed communication activities of people with aphasia and healthy older people. Paper presented at International Aphasia Rehabilitation Conference, September, Johannesburg, South Africa.

Davis GA, Wilcox MJ (1985). Adult Aphasia Rehabilitation: Applied Pragmatics. Windsor: NFER-Nelson.

Elman R (1998). Memories of the 'plateau': health-care changes provide an opportunity to redefine aphasia treatment and discharge. Aphasiology 12(3): 227–31.

Elman R, Bernstein-Ellis E (1995). What is functional? American Journal of Speech-Language Pathology 4: 115–17.

Finkelstein V, French S (1993). Towards a psychology of disability. In Swain J, Finkelstein V, French S, Oliver M (eds) Disabling barriers – Enabling Environments. London: Open University Publications and Sage, pp.26–33.

Goodwin C (1995). Co-constructing meaning in conversations with an aphasic man. In Jacoby E, Ochs E (eds) Research on Language and Social Interaction (Special issue on co-construction), pp.233–60.

Helm-Estabrooks N, Ramsberger G (1986). Treatment of agrammatism in long-term Broca's aphasia. British Journal of Disorders of Communication 211(1): 39–45.

Holland A (1982). Observing functional communication in aphasic adults. Journal of Speech and Hearing Disorders 47: 50–6.

Holland A (1991). Pragmatic aspects of intervention in aphasia. Journal of Neurolinguistics 6: 197–211.

Holland AL, Beeson PM (1999). In Elman R (ed.) Group Treatment of Neurogenic Communication Disorders. Boston, MA: Butterworth Heinemann, pp.77–84.

Hughes K, Paterson G (1997). The social model of disability and the disappearing body: towards a sociology of impairment. Disability and Society 12(3): 325–40.

Ireland C (1995). 100 years on from Freud's 'On Aphasia': from patient to counsellor. In Code C, Muller D (eds) The Treatment of Aphasia: From Theory to Practice. London: Whurr Publishers, pp.29–43.

Ireland C, Wootton G (1996). Time to talk. Disability and Rehabilitation 18: 585–91.

Jones E (1986). Building the foundations for sentence production in a non-fluent aphasic. British Journal of Disorders of Communication 21(1): 63–82.

Joseph Rowntree Foundation (1995). Building Social Capital in a 21st Century Welfare State. York: Joseph Rowntree Foundation.

Kagan A (1995). Revealing the competence of aphasic adults through conversation: a challenge to health professionals. Topics in Stroke Rehabilitation 2(1): 15–28.

Kagan A (1998). Supported conversation for adults with aphasia: methods and resources for training conversation partners. Aphasiology 12: 816–30.

Kagan A, Gailey G (1993). Functional is not enough: training conversation partners for aphasic adults. In Holland A, Forbes M (eds) Aphasia Treatment: World Perspectives. San Diego, CA: Singular Press, pp.199-225.

Kleinman A (1988). The Illness Narratives: Suffering, Healing and the Human Condition. New York: Harper Collins.

Lafond D, JoanetteY, Ponzio J, Degiovani R, Taylor Sarno M (eds) (1993). Living with Aphasia: Psychosocial Issues. San Diego, CA: Singular Press.

Lesser R, Algar L (1995). Towards combining the cognitive neuropsychological and the pragmatic in aphasia therapy. Neuropsychological Rehabilitation 5(1/2): 67–92.

Levenson R, Farrell C (1998). Public Health and the PAMS. London: King's Fund Institute.

Lyon J (1997). Coping with Aphasia. San Diego, CA: Singular Press.

Lyon J (1998). Treating real life functionality in a couple coping with severe aphasia. In Helm-Estabrooks N, Holland A (eds) Approaches to Treatment in Aphasia. San Diego, CA: Singular Press, pp.203–39.

Lyon J, Cariski D, Keisler L, Rosenbek J, Levine R, Kumpula J, Ryff C, Coyne S, Levine J (1997). Communication partners: enhancing participation in life and communication for adults with aphasia in natural settings. Aphasiology 11: 693–708.

Marshall J, Pring TR, Chiat S (1993). Sentence processing therapy – working at the level of the event. Aphasiology 7(2): 177–99.

McCrae Cochrane R, Milton S (1984). Conversational prompting: a sentence building technique for severe aphasia. Journal of Neurological Communication Disorders 1: 4–23.

Nichols F, Varchevker A, Pring T (1996). Working with people with aphasia and their families: an exploration of the use of family therapy techniques. Aphasiology 10(8): 767–81.

Oliver M (1996). Understanding Disability: From Theory to Practice. Basingstoke and London: Macmillan.

Parr S, Byng S, Gilpin S (1997). Talking about Aphasia: Living with Loss of Language after Stroke. Buckingham: Open University Press.

Parr S, Pound C, Byng S, Long B (1999). The Aphasia Handbook. London: Connect Press.

Penman T (1998). Self advocacy and aphasia. Bulletin of the Royal College of Speech and Language Therapists 556: 14–15.

Peters S (1996). The politics of disability identity. In Barton L (ed.) Disability and Society: Emerging Issues and Insights. London and New York: Longman, pp.215–37.

Pound C (1998). Power, partnerships and perspectives: social model approaches to long term aphasia therapy and support. Paper presented at the 8th International Aphasia Rehabilitation Conference, Pilanesburg, South Africa.

Pound C, Parr S, Clarke M (1998) Caring and coping in long term aphasia: in-depth interviewing as a tool for revealing the benefits and limitations of relative support groups. Poster presented at the 8th International Aphasia Rehabilitation Conference, Pilanesburg, South Africa.

Rice B, Paull A, Muller D (1987). An evaluation of a social support group for spouses of aphasic partners. Aphasiology 1(3): 247–56.

Rucker C (1998). Clinical Portfolio, Advanced Clinical Studies Certificate, City University, London.

Sacchett C, Byng S, Marshall J, Pound C (1999). Drawing together: evaluation of a therapy programme for severe aphasia. International Journal of Disorders of Language and Communication 34(3): 265–89.

Sacks O (1984, 1991). A Leg to Stand on. London: Pan Books.

Sarno MT (1993). Aphasia rehabilitation: psychosocial and ethical considerations. Aphasiology 7: 321–34.

Simmons N (1993). An Ethnographic Investigation of Compensatory Strategies in Aphasia. Dissertation, Louisiana State University and Agricultural and Mechanical College, Louisiana, USA.

Simmons-Mackie N, Damico JS (1997). Reformulating the definition of compensatory strategies in aphasia. Aphasiology 11(8): 761–81.

Smith L (1985). Communicative activities of dysphasic adults: a survey. British Journal of Disorders of Communication 20: 31–44.

Starkstein SE, Robinson RG (1988). Aphasia and depression. Aphasiology 2: 1–20.

Tanner D, Gerstenberger D (1988). The grief response in neuropathologies of speech and language. Aphasiology 2: 79–84.

Thompson CK, Shapiro LP, Roberts MM (1993). Treatment of sentence production deficits in aphasia: a linguistic-specific approach to wh-interrogative training and generalisation. Aphasiology 7: 111–33.

Wahrborg P, Borenstein P (1989). Family therapy in families with an aphasic member. Aphasiology 3(1): 93–7.

Chapter 4
Cognitive neuropsychology and aphasia therapy: the case of word retrieval

DAVID HOWARD

Cognitive neuropsychology

Twenty-five years after the publication of Marshall and Newcombe's famous paper 'Patterns of paralexia' (1973), it is hard to see it as ground-breaking. What then could be seen as innovations – and which were, at that time, almost shocking – now seem simply commonplace. In the paper Marshall and Newcombe analysed the reading performance of three single subjects with acquired reading disorders. They showed that the patients had qualitatively different impairments, and that these impairments could be understood in terms of an information-processing model derived from normal subjects' performance. In that paper, they coined the terms *deep dyslexia*, *surface dyslexia* and *visual dyslexia*. The first two of these have become the common currency of any contemporary classification of the dyslexias. The other feature that was novel for a neuropsychological paper at the time was that Marshall and Newcombe had nothing to say about the localization of function in the brain – their argument was in terms of processing models not cerebral structures.

Cognitive neuropsychology was slow to start. 'Patterns of paralexia' was published in 1973, and although there was a trickle of papers in the intervening years, the real landmark, establishing the approach, was the publication of the book *Deep Dyslexia* edited by Coltheart, Patterson and Marshall in 1980. This now reads almost as a manifesto for a new way of doing neuropsychology – an approach that aimed at understanding the details of individual patients' behaviour from principled scientific modelling.

The journal *Cognitive Neuropsychology* was launched in 1984, with a trenchant editorial by Max Coltheart, arguing that data from single subjects were the only productive way of using neuropsychological data to understand normal cognitive systems (Coltheart, 1984).

Since then, the approach has been extremely successful. Cognitive neuropsychological approaches have developed a great deal of diversity, expanding from an initial interest in reading and other language disorders to almost all areas of cognitive disorders – perception (the agnosias), semantic, episodic and short-term memory, and disorders of action, drawing, planning, and so on. They have been so successful that *Cognitive Neuropsychology* is the most cited journal in cognitive psychology, and among the most cited experimental psychology journals.

The distinguishing feature of cognitive neuropsychology is, then, an interest in investigating and understanding single subjects; single subjects are the focus of interest, because it is impossible *a priori* to be sure that two different subjects have the same underlying deficits (Caramazza, 1984). These deficits are identified using converging evidence from the variables affecting performance, relative accuracy in different tasks, and the types of errors. Cognitive neuropsychologists have generally been uninterested in explanations at neurological levels rather than in terms of information-processing models; this partly reflects the way that cognitive neuropsychology was a reaction to the neuropsychology of the 1950s–1970s in which, at least in caricature, the purpose was to locate symptoms in terms of brain structures on the basis of group, lesion-defined data. More recently, there has been a trend towards greater interest in the cortical mechanisms underlying cognitive function, fuelled principally by the potential for localizing cognitive functions offered by PET (positron emission tomography) and, more recently, fMRI (functional magnetic resonance imaging) (see Frith and Friston, 1997; Howard, 1997; Price, 1997).

Cognitive neuropsychology and the assessment of naming

In this chapter I will consider the contribution of cognitive neuropsychology to the clinical assessment and treatment of aphasic disorders of word retrieval. Cognitive neuropsychologists have used models of word retrieval which distinguish between a number of different stages in word retrieval. The distinction between these stages is motivated in part by experimental work with normal subjects, but these models have also drawn support from neuropsychological studies of brain-damaged patients. An outline model is shown in Figure 4.1. The hypothesis is that each level of processing can be selectively impaired by acquired brain damage, and that the level of deficit can be identified on the basis of converging evidence from (i) the patient's performance in different tasks which tap representations at that and other levels, (ii) the effects of different psycholinguistic variables, such as word concreteness, length or frequency on patients' performance, and (iii) the nature of the errors that a patient makes in word comprehension and production. The conjunction of evidence of these different kinds can be used to determine the patient's level of breakdown. Then, in turn, the demonstration that the model can be used successfully to characterize a patient's deficit increases confidence in the model's explanatory adequacy.

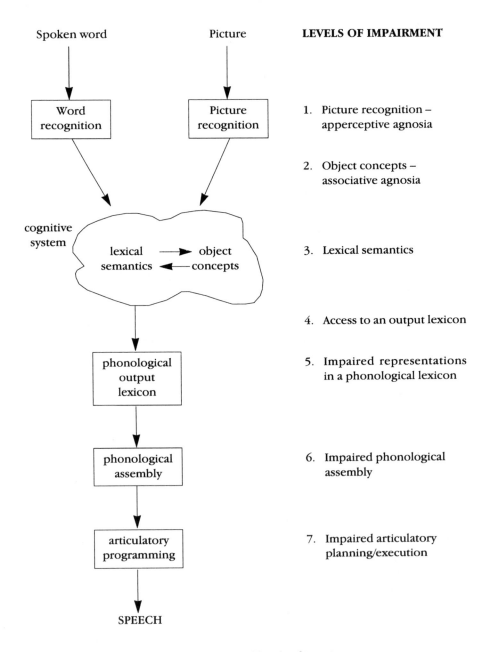

Figure 4.1: A simple model of naming, and levels of impairment.

Table 4.1 summarizes current knowledge of the nature of deficits at different levels and their characteristic features. A detailed description and defence of this model is beyond the scope of this chapter (see Nickels and Howard (in press) for recent review). Two examples will be described briefly:

(1) Semantic impairment

Patients with central lexical semantic impairments make errors in both comprehension and production of words (for example, Howard and Orchard-Lisle, 1984; Caramazza and Hillis, 1990). That the impairment affects only lexical semantic representations, while non-linguistic conceptual representations are intact, is demonstrated by, for instance, Howard and Orchard-Lisle's (1984) patient JCU's intact performance in the picture version of the Pyramids and Palm Trees Test. That the lexical-semantic representations are impaired, and, specifically, are underspecified – in the sense that they specify the category to which an item belongs but not the specific target word – is demonstrated by the finding that these subjects benefit from correct phonemic cues, but are induced to make semantic errors by miscues – cues using the initial phoneme of a coordinate member of the semantic category. These patients make predominantly semantically related errors in naming and their naming accuracy is affected primarily by the concreteness, or imageability of the target name (Nickels and Howard, 1994; Nickels, 1995).

(2) Post-lexical impairment in phonological assembly

An impairment in post-lexical phonological assembly is completely different. These patients have increasing rates of error with longer words – word length affects both the complexity of, and the opportunity for, errors in phonological assembly (Caplan, Vanier and Baker, 1986; Nickels and Howard, 1995). Their errors are phonologically related to the target, showing that they are based on access to the correct entry in the phonological output lexicon. That these entries have been correctly accessed can be demonstrated by showing that these patients can make correct judgements about the phonological form even of words that they cannot produce, in, for instance, picture homophone judgements (Feinberg, Rothi and Heilman, 1986). In addition to these features, which are consistent with a deficit in the process of phonological assembly, these patients typically do not show the features of a semantic level of impairment. That is, naming accuracy is unaffected by semantic properties such as word concreteness or semantic category. True, semantic errors do not occur, but patients sometimes produce circumlocutory descriptions when unable to produce a target word.

Table 4.1: Levels of impairment and their characteristics: a summary

Level of impairment	Sometimes known as	Naming error types	Factors affecting naming accuracy	Other features
Picture recognition	Apperceptive agnosia	Mostly visually related	Visual complexity effect. May be better with inanimate than animate items. Naming to touch or definition better than picture naming	Word comprehension typically good, although not when tested with picture materials
Object concepts	Associative agnosia/ semantic dementia	Semantic errors (often superordinates).	Typically large frequency effects. May show semantic category effects	Word comprehension is poor. Poor performance in semantic judgments with pictures.
Lexical semantics		Semantic errors.	Imageability/concreteness effects possible. No effects of word length. Phonemic cues and miscues may have an effect.	Good at picture semantics but impaired in word comprehension.
Access to an output lexicon	Classical anomia (?)	Error types uncertain: semantic errors or no responses.	Naming should be improved by a correct phonemic cue. Inconsistent	Comprehension good.
Impaired representations in a phonological lexicon		Errors should be descriptions etc. and ? strategic semantic errors	Consistent. Frequency/familiarity effect. No effects of semantic or phonological variables.	Comprehension good.
Impaired phonological assembly	Conduction aphasia (?)	Errors should be primarily phonological	Length effect (poorer with longer words) Difficulty in naming, reading and repetition should be similar. Written output better. Probably a frequency effect, Better with real words than non-words. Probably should be good at tests of phonological knowledge.	Comprehension should be good.
Impaired articulatory programming/ execution	Articulatory apraxia/ dysarthria	Phonologically/ articulatorily related errors	Effects of length, articulatory complexity and probably stress pattern. No lexical or semantic variables affect performance. Written naming should be better.	Comprehension good.

These examples illustrate how mappings can be made between features of aphasic word retrieval and levels of impairment in terms of an information-processing model. While this mapping gives real confidence that the distinctions between processing levels capture important properties of the processes in word retrieval, at the same time these models are both a simplification and a partial description. They are a simplification in the sense that some of the boxes and arrows in these models may themselves be decomposable into further processes. For example, a considerable body of data now converges on the conclusion that the process of mapping from a semantic representation to lexical phonological forms involves, as an intermediate stage, retrieval of a word-specific lemma (see Levelt (1989); Levelt et al. (1999) for data from normal subjects, and Nickels and Howard (in press) for neuropsychological arguments).

This model is also a partial description in the sense that the details of the processes carried out within the boxes are not specified in any detail. It is likely, for example, that the process of phonological assembly involves generation of a CV frame (specifying the consonant–vowel sequence), insertion of segments into the frame, and the process of generation of a prosodic contour (see also Levelt, 1989).

This kind of assessment schema has obvious appeal for clinicians. First, the proposal of quite distinct levels of breakdown accords with clinical experience of quite different types of word-finding difficulty. Second, the different features associated with different levels of breakdown translate easily into assessment procedures that can identify different levels of breakdown. Third, use of these assessment procedures allows clinicians to identify both impaired and intact processing components giving crucial information both about levels that should be targeted in treatment and the resources that can be used in treatment.

Treatment of word retrieval deficits

It has often been pointed out that identifying a particular level of breakdown does not, of itself, identify the optimal kind of treatment (see Howard and Hatfield, 1987; Behrmann and Byng, 1992; Caramazza and Hillis, 1993). However, at a first approximation, cognitive neuropsychological approaches to treatment invite the idea that it might be empirically possible, using a series of studies of treatment effects with individual patients, to identify the optimal treatment strategy for a patient with a particular type of impairment. Notice that the claim that there are different levels of impairment in word retrieval does not *necessarily* mean that different kinds of treatment will be appropriate: it might, for instance, be the case that the best kind of treatment for all levels of breakdown in word retrieval might be practice in saying a target word. The cognitive neuropsychological approach offers: (i) the possibility that treatment effectiveness will be related to level of breakdown, and (ii) the possibility that treatment designed on the basis of knowledge of intact and impaired processes will be most effective. It seems likely that both of these are true, but whether they are is an empirical question.

Semantic versus phonological facilitation

One approach to understanding the process of treatment is to study the effects of single treatment events on patients' ability to retrieve words. Howard et al. (1985a) argued that one could distinguish between three kinds of effects: see Table 4.2. The immediate effects of prompts on word retrieval have been widely studied in group and individual studies. In general, phonemic cues, the first sound or the first syllable of a target word, are very effective cues to word retrieval (for example, Pease and Goodglass, 1978), although these effects are not found for all subjects (for example, Bruce and Howard, 1988). In contrast, semantic cues, which provide the patient with some information about the meaning of the target item – typically its category or some attribute – are relatively ineffective, probably because this conceptual information is what the patients already have.

Table 4.2: Prompting, facilitation and therapy: the distinction

Prompting
When a patient cannot name a picture, the therapist applies a technique *once*.
Effect measured as the difference in naming accuracy *immediately* after prompting, relative to uncued control items

Facilitation
When a patient cannot name a picture, the therapist applies a technique *once*.
Effect measured as the difference in naming accuracy for treated items relative to untreated controls *at some later time* – 5 minutes, 24 hours or 2 weeks later. Facilitation is the long-term effect of a single technique used once.

Therapy
Describes the *multiple use* of (usually) a variety of techniques to try to effect a *long-term change* in a patient's ability to retrieve a word.
Effect measured as either (a) accuracy in naming treated items relative to untreated controls after treatment, or (b) improvement for treated items relative to pre-treatment naming.

Studies of prompting effects show that phonemic information about a target word is an effective cue. An influential paper by Patterson, Purell and Morton (1983) showed that these effects, while large, disappeared rapidly. In two experiments they demonstrated that: (i) having repeated a word makes it accessible as a picture name temporarily, but the effect disappears within 5–10 minutes, and (ii) having been phonemically cued to produce a target word does not affect the likelihood that the picture can be correctly named 25 minutes later.

The short-lasting effects of these techniques, which provide information about the phonological form of a sought-for word, can be contrasted with a set of techniques that do not involve production of the target word. In a series of experiments, Howard et al. (1985a) showed that any technique which requires the patient to access the semantics corresponding to the picture name results in facilitation of word retrieval which lasts for at least 30 minutes, and, in the experiments where this was tested, the effects were still apparent, and undiminished, after 24 hours (see Figure 4.2). Similar effects were found from: auditory word-to-picture matching (point to one of four pictures when its name is spoken by the examiner); visual word-to-picture matching; and semantic judgements (answer a yes/no question about the meaning of a picture name (for example, 'does a cow eat grass?')). This long-term facilitation effect does not, therefore, require saying the word, hearing the word or seeing the target picture.

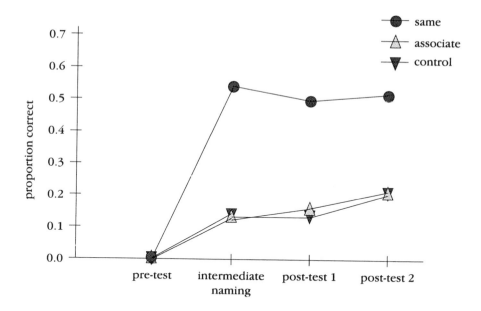

Figure 4.2: The accuracy of picture naming following different cueing conditions measured at intermediate naming (2–3 minutes after facilitation), post-test 1 (about 30 minutes after facilitation), and post-test 2 (24 hours later). The facilitation conditions are (when *lion* is not named in the pre-test): (i) 'Same' – word-to-picture matching for the target picture (for example, target '*lion*', choices *tiger, lion, elephant, giraffe*); (ii) 'Associate' – word-to-picture matching for a closely associated coordinate (for example, target '*tiger*', choices *tiger, lion, elephant, giraffe*); (iii) 'Control' – no facilitation. Improvement in naming relative to the control condition is only found when the target word is used in word-to-picture matching. Figure adapted from Howard et al. (1985a).

It seems unlikely that the comprehension tasks are in any sense providing semantic information about the target names, for two reasons. First, the priming effects were found equally for subjects who performed normally in the Pyramids and Palm Trees test (a non-verbal test of conceptual semantics; Howard and Patterson, 1992), and those that performed poorly (suggesting that these subjects' conceptual representations may have been degraded). Second, these treatment effects were found even though the treatment task was very easy and carried out accurately by almost all the subjects (Franklin, 1993). On the basis of these findings, Howard et al. (1985a) argue that these effects were priming of a word-specific lexical semantic representation. Access to semantics in the comprehension task primed a lemma representation; this primed lemma was then more easily accessible when the picture was subsequently presented for naming.

Subsequent work on these semantic facilitation effects are consistent with this interpretation. Barry and McHattie (1991) confirmed these facilitation effects and went on to show that they were unrelated to the detail involved in the semantic judgement. They found equal facilitation of naming from answering a question requiring only access to superficial category semantic information (for example, 'Is a duck or a train a living thing?'), a question requiring access to intermediate semantic information ('Is a duck or a cat a bird?'), and one requiring access to precise item-specific semantics ('Is a swan or a duck a water bird with webbed feet and which quacks?'). Le Dorze et al. (1994) showed that the target lexical item was required; while 'Show me the octopus' primed naming, 'Show me the mollusc with long legs' did not.

While long-lasting semantic effects have been found, it is less than completely clear that phonological treatments truly have only short-lasting effects. Barry and McHattie (1991), for example, found that repetition of a target name resulted in significant improvement in naming when pictures were presented for naming about 10-15 minutes later, and significant measurable effects, when the probe of naming performance was delayed for a further thirty minutes. This finding cannot be easily reconciled with Patterson et al's finding that phonological facilitation effects are very short-lasting.

Semantic and phonological therapy

The finding that a single semantic task could improve the accessibility of a target word for at least 24 hours, in contrast to phonological techniques, which have only short-lasting effects, prompted the first systematic use of these tasks in treatment.

Howard et al. (1985b) compared daily treatment of two sets of target items with phonological and semantic treatments, given over separate time periods. The semantic treatment consisted of spoken and written word-to-picture matching and semantic judgements, and the phonological therapy comprised word repetition, phonemic cueing and rhyme judgements. Twelve subjects were treated for either 1 or 2 weeks with each of these techniques.

Performance on the treated items was probed every day during therapy at the beginning of each session, 24 hours after the last session, and again 1 week and 6 weeks after treatment had finished, and finally at the end of the experiment. In addition to the treated items, there were naming controls, which were presented for naming as often as the treated items, but were never treated. These were to control for the possibility that opportunities for naming were responsible for any improvement. In addition there were baseline controls which were presented for naming only in the pre- and post-therapy tests and never appeared during the treatment period.

Howard et al. reported that, across their 12 subjects, both treatment techniques resulted in improvements in naming, with day-by-day improvements which were greater for treated items than naming controls – items that were presented for naming as often as treated items, but never themselves treated (see Figure 4.3). Using analysis of variance, they examined the effects of semantic and phonological treatments 1 and 6 weeks after treatment, comparing treated items with their naming controls and baseline controls (see Table 4.3). They concluded that, 1 week after treatment, there were significant advantages for treated items relative to controls, but that the advantages were only significant 1 week after treatment ended. There was a significant, but small advantage for semantic treatment over phonological treatment, primarily evident in better performance with semantic naming controls.

Recent reanalysis using more focused statistical techniques suggest that the original conclusions were rather pessimistic. Combining across the treatment techniques, treated items are named better than baseline controls at 1 week, 6 weeks and at the end of the experiment (combined S test, $p=0.002$ or better; see Table 4.3). Treated items are also named better than their naming controls at the end of treatment (combined S test, $z=4.21$, $p<0.001$), 1 week ($z=2.50$, $p=0.006$) and 6 weeks later ($z=1.82$, $p=0.034$), although the difference was no longer significant at the end of the whole experiment (that is, 7 weeks after the last treatment block; $z=0.44$, ns). The differences between the two techniques are minimal: the only significant effect is for better performance with semantic naming controls than phonological naming controls 1 week after therapy.

There are also no differences between the treatments as measured by performance in the daily pre-tests during the period of therapy. The rates of improvement are significantly different from zero for all sets of items involved in treatment (semantic items, $t(11)=3.86$, semantic naming controls, $t(11)=3.11$, phonological items, $t(11)=5.67$, phonological

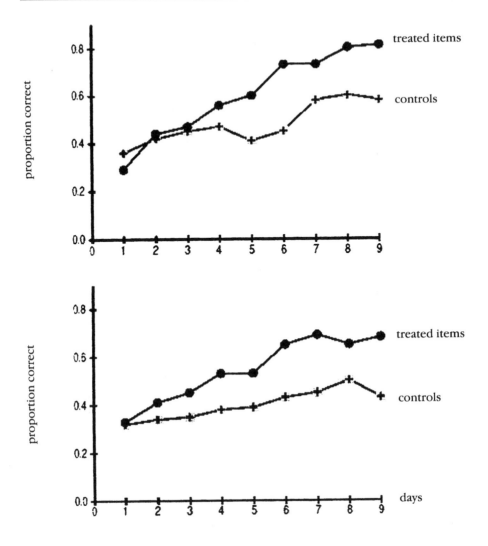

Figure 4.3: Naming of pictures during two therapy periods as measured in pre-tests before treatment on each day. Naming controls were presented for naming as often as treatment items but never treated. Redrawn from Howard et al. (1985b).

naming controls, $t(11)=2.87$; $p<0.01$ in all cases), and these gradients are greater for treated items than the naming controls (semantic $t(11)=3.28$, phonological $t(11)=2.04$, $p<0.05$), but there is no difference in the rate of improvement for the two types of therapy (treated items $t(11)=1.25$, ns, naming controls $t(11)=-0.23$, ns).

These analyses address only the questions of whether, on average, over the group of patients, the semantic and phonological treatments were effective, and whether, on average, there was a difference between the effectiveness of the two types of treatment. The finding that both

Table 4.3: The performance on treated items, naming controls and baseline controls, 24 hours after treatment, 1 week after treatment, 6 weeks after treatment, and at the end of the experiment (7 or 13 weeks after treatment). Data from 12 patients, half treated for 1 week and half for 2 weeks with each therapy method. (Based on Howard et al., 1985b)

Naming accuracy for:	Interval after treatment			
	24 hrs	1 week	6 weeks	End
Semantic therapy treated items	0.621	0.550	0.458	0.450
Semantic naming controls	0.475	0.492	0.392	0.442
Semantic baseline controls	–	0.383	0.333	0.342
Phonological therapy treated items	0.577	0.500	0.446	0.425
Phonological naming controls	0.408	0.375	0.375	0.400
Phonological baseline controls	–	0.329	0.396	0.342

treatments were, essentially, equally effective is, however, consistent with two quite distinct possibilities. One is that, across the group of subjects, the semantic and phonological treatment effects were equal – patients who benefited from one treatment also improved with the other. The other possibility, which has very different implications, is that some of the patients benefited from the semantic treatments, and others – perhaps those with problems primarily concerning post-lexical difficulties in word production – benefit from the phonological treatments.

Once reanalysed, the data from the experiment are quite clear. Five of the 12 patients show no evidence at any point of benefiting from either therapy method. These patients cannot contribute any information about relative effectiveness of the treatments, because, for them, both methods were ineffective. The remaining seven patients provide unequivocal results. There is a very high correlation between the rate of improvement during the two types of therapy ($r=0.882$). Similarly, there is a high correlation between naming accuracy on the items treated by the two methods at the end of therapy ($r=0.820$) and after 1 week ($r=0.905$). A homogeneity test on the difference between the effects of the two treatments confirms that there are no substantial differences in their relative effectiveness. In essence, these results show that patients who responded better to the phonological treatments also responded best to the semantic treatments, and that there was no evidence that any patient benefited more from one treatment than the other.

Why might this be? There are, essentially, two different possibilities. The first is that, as Howard et al. (1985b) suggested, when intensive, daily treatment of word retrieval is used, the nature of that treatment does not matter very much. The second is that the two treatment techniques provide very similar information, although in slightly different ways. Both provide the patient with information about – and practice in – the mapping from meaning to lexical phonological representation.

Semantic therapy

A number of subsequent studies have shown that 'semantic' therapy, based on the facilitation techniques shown to be effective, can have long-lasting but generally item-specific effects in improving word retrieval.

For example, Marshall and colleagues (1990) treated seven patients who had better word reading than picture naming. During the treatment period, the subjects had to match one of four written words to a picture. One of the written words was the target name, two were semantically related and one was unrelated. The patients made these judgements twice a day, 5 days a week over 2 weeks. Naming was probed at the end of treatment, 1 month later, and for six of the seven subjects, a year after treatment (Pring et al., 1990). In addition to the treated items, performance was assessed on two other sets of items: 'related' items that had appeared as semantically related distractors in the word-to-picture matching task, but had not been target names; and 'seen' items that were unrelated distractors in matching, and 'unseen' controls that had not appeared during the treatment phase. The results of this study are summarized in Figure 4.4. There was significant improvement only for the treated items relative to the unseen controls. The limited amount of treatment, however, resulted in treatment effects which were still apparent a year after the treatment ended.

These results accord with those found by Howard et al. (1985b); limited amounts of treatment result in long-term changes in the

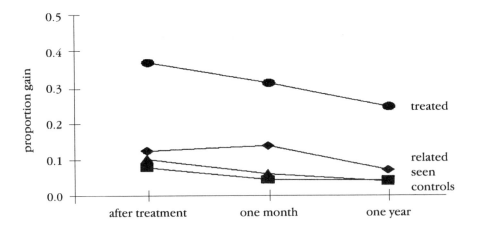

Figure 4.4: Treatment by Marshall et al. (1990) of seven patients by written word-to-picture matching. Naming was assessed on treated items, related distracters in word-to-picture matching, 'seen' items (unrelated distracters from word-to-picture matching) and 'unseen' controls, immediately following treatment (which lasted for two weeks), one month and one year later. There is significant improvement relative to 'unseen' controls for the treated items at all post-therapy tests.

patients' ability to retrieve target words, but the effects are, essentially, limited to the items that are targeted in treatment.

Evidence for any generalization has been hard to find in these kinds of 'semantic' therapies. The only group study of patients finding generalization is by Pring and colleagues (1993). They studied the performance of subjects in naming items from a set of semantic categories. There were two therapy tasks: in the first, subjects had to decide which of four written words was the name of a single picture, with all the words drawn from the same category as the target. In the second therapy task, six pictures were presented with three written words, which were the names of target, treated items. All the pictures were drawn from one semantic category. Treatment took place over 10 sessions spread over 2 weeks; each target item was treated twice with one of the two techniques in each session. Performance was tested before treatment, afterwards and 1 month later on four sets of items: treated items, related seen items (whose names and pictures had appeared as distracters during treatment), related unseen items (other items from the same semantic categories as the targets and the related seen items, which had never appeared in the treatment task), and control items (which were from a different semantic category, and had never occurred during treatment). The results are shown in Figure 4.5.

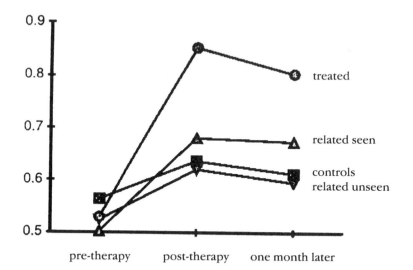

Figure 4.5: Proportion correct in naming for treated items, related seen items (semantically related distractors from word-to-picture matching), related unseen items (semantically related items not occurring during therapy) and unseen control items, before and after treatment and one month later. There is significant improvement for treated items relative to controls and limited, but statistically significant, improvement with 'related seen' items. Results are from five patients after two weeks of treatment. Drawn from data given by Pring, Hamilton, Harwood and Macbride (1993).

After treatment, performance on the treated items and on the related seen items is significantly better than on the controls and the related unseen items, which did not differ. The related seen items have improved, but to a much smaller extent than the treated items. This experiment, then, shows a limited degree of generalization to related distracters which appeared during the therapy tasks. However, as I shall argue in the next section, on at least one interpretation, this is not a true generalization effect, but a treatment effect.

Towards an account of treatment effects

Suppose that the treatment effects are due to strengthening of the mapping between meaning representations and the phonological word forms, and that these mappings are strengthened when the semantic and phonological representations are simultaneously active. This clearly happens during the therapy tasks where the patients were asked to read the target names aloud and choose the appropriate picture or the appropriate name. The extent to which the patients complied with the instruction to read the words aloud is unclear, as, in this experiment, much of the treatment was unsupervised. However, this probably does not matter; there is abundant evidence that when comprehending written words normal subjects automatically activate words' phonological representations (for example, Van Orden, Johnston and Hale, 1988; Coltheart, Patterson and Leahy, 1994). This presumably, also applies to aphasic patients, at least to the extent that they can activate the phonology. It is also clear that the semantics of these written words will be activated; the treatment task requires semantic processing to reject them as inappropriate picture names. Thus, to the extent that the treatment task involves simultaneous activation of semantics and phonology for the 'related seen' items, they are being treated. Presumably, they benefit less from treatment than the treated items because less attention may have been paid to processing the items, at least after some practice with the task.

This hypothesis would also account for the pattern of results in the Howard et al. (1985b) study. Here, items treated both with phonological therapy and semantic therapy improved, and to a lesser extent there was improvement with naming controls which were repeatedly presented for naming without any specific treatment. Treatment of both kinds involves simultaneous activation of semantic and phonological representations for the target items. Although the semantic treatments did not require overt production of the target during word-to-picture matching, there is, again, abundant evidence that, with normal subjects (and also, probably, aphasic patients), hearing or seeing a word results in automatic activation of both semantics and output phonology (for example, Shriefers et al., 1990). The improvement with naming controls can be accounted for in a similar way. The pictures were repeatedly presented for naming, but without help. When, by chance, a subject managed to produce a target name, both the semantic representation and the phonological representation were simultaneously active. This then strengthens the mapping for that item, making it more likely that the word will be produced correctly on a subsequent occasion (which will again strengthen the mapping). This predicts that repeated presentation will result in progressive improvements in naming; a finding that Nickels and Best (in press) report.

The facilitation results reported earlier could be accounted for by the same hypothesis. Thus, all the semantic tasks that Howard et al. (1985a) and Barry and McHattie (1991) found to be effective, long-term facilitators of word retrieval involve simultaneous activation of semantics and phonology, if we accept that words which are heard or seen automatically activate output phonology. The difficulty with this account is the Patterson et al. (1983) findings that neither word repetition nor phonemic cueing resulted in any long-term facilitation. Both of these tasks also involve simultaneous activation of semantics and phonology. It is possible to argue that the failure to find a facilitation effect from repetition may partly be because there was a long list of items repeated without any semantic context; this may have encouraged the patients to approach the task as one of word reproduction minimizing the semantic processing. Barry and McHattie's (1991) finding that word repetition did result in some longer-term facilitation of word retrieval supports this possibility. The failure to find facilitation from phonemic cueing, despite considerable correct name retrieval immediately following the cue, remains a problem.

If the hypothesis put forward here is correct, the 'semantic therapy' effects found in the studies by Howard et al. (1985b) and by Pring and his colleagues are not, in any real sense, semantic. That is, the treatment is not effective because it allows patients to access more detailed, 'better' semantics for naming. In discussing the facilitation results, I argued that there were several lines of evidence that made this hypothesis unlikely. The therapy studies yield one result supporting this conclusion. If semantic therapies were having their effects at a semantic level, the treatment should be primarily effective for subjects with a semantic impairment. Pring, Davis and Marshall (1993) examined whether the amount of improvement in their semantic therapy experiments was related to patients' ability to access the semantics of words and pictures. All the correlations were positive – that is, improvement was greater for patients who did *better* at the comprehension tasks, and the correlation was significant for the Pyramids and Palm Trees Test (Howard and Patterson, 1992). That is the patients with *less* semantic impairment in judging whether pictures were related made the *most* improvement – a result very difficult to reconcile with any hypothesis that semantic therapy was effective at a semantic level.

The suggestion that the treatment effects result from improvement – strengthening – of the mapping from semantics to phonology also provides a simple account of why these treatment effects are item-specific and do not generalize. The mappings from meaning to lexical form are almost wholly arbitrary. Words with similar meanings do not have similar phonological forms; knowing that one kind of pet is called a *dog* is of no help in knowing that another is a *cat*. Because the mapping is arbitrary and item-specific, we would not expect true generalization.

Lexical therapy

Some recent studies have examined the effects of 'lexical' therapy (for example, Miceli et al., 1996; Nickels and Best, 1996b). In essence, these approaches intend to improve the mapping from meaning to sound directly, with patients who show intact semantics and impairment to naming as a result of a difficulty in access to lexical representations, or, possibly, impairment to the phonological representations.

Miceli and colleagues (1996) describe treatment results with two rather similar patients. One, GMA, will be taken as an example. He was poor at naming, and nearly all of his errors were no responses or circumlocutions. His comprehension of words was very good, including the names of pictures which he could not name. This pattern of performance led Miceli et al. to conclude that GMA's deficit was at the level of the output lexicon.

Three different therapy methods were used with three different sets of pictures. Each treatment was carried out daily for a week, and naming of the whole set was tested before and after each treatment period. A fourth set of items acted as controls, and were never treated. The treatment methods used were:

(i)   Picture + reading: given the picture and its written name; read the name.
(ii) Reading: read aloud the written word.
(iii) Picture alone: given the picture to name, and then given progressive phonemic cues until the correct name was retrieved.

The results are shown in Figure 4.6, top panel. Each set improved to almost 100% correct in the week in which it was treated, but in each period there was no improvement in untreated items. Naming performance was probed repeatedly over the following 17 months (see Figure 4.6, bottom panel). The advantage for the treated items was sustained, although somewhat reduced, over the whole 17-month period.

The results of this experiment, and others using lexical therapy by Nickels and Best (1996b), show that substantial and long-lasting, item-specific improvement can be made with small amounts of treatment, which emphasize, basically, learning the phonological word form that goes with the picture.

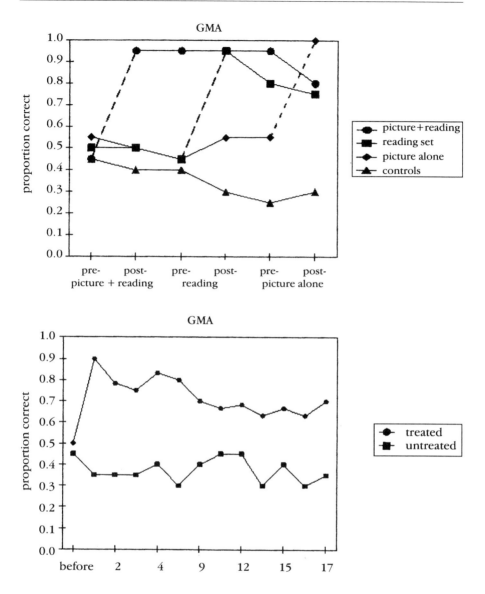

Figure 4.6: Top panel: This shows the results of lexical therapy by three different treatment methods for GMA. The period when treatment was applied for each set is shown be dashed lines. Bottom panel: This shows naming accuracy for treated and control items probed at various periods over the 17 months after treatment ended. Drawn from data given by Miceli et al. (1996).

It should be clear, however, that 'lexical' therapy may not be different, in any important way, from 'semantic' therapy or 'phonological' therapy. All of these techniques provide simultaneous activation of phonological and semantic representations. The differences between these techniques may be more apparent than real.

Treatment with strategies

All the treatments described so far produce item-specific effects. I have argued, indeed, that the cases of supposed 'generalization' are not really generalization (in the sense that improvements on target items themselves directly result in improvements with items not explicitly targeted). The 'generalization' described represents only item-specific treatment effects occurring during therapy, which were not the target of treatment. That treatment effects are item-specific is a simple consequence of the arbitrary mapping from semantics to phonology.

Generalization can be anticipated only from treatment techniques that provide the patients with a general strategy for aiding the mapping from semantics to phonology.

For example, Bruce and Howard (1987) describe a treatment approach where patients used a computer to convert the initial letter of a target name into a phonemic cue. They worked with five patients who had relatively accurate knowledge of the initial letter of a target name which they could not name, and who benefited from phonemic cues given by the therapist. None of these subjects had any knowledge of letter-to-sound correspondences. Rather than teaching the patients letter-to-sound correspondences, which can be a lengthy and laborious process (Berman and Peelle, 1967; de Partz, 1986), Bruce and Howard taught the patients to use the computer prosthesis over four weekly sessions. After treatment the patients were tested on 100 pictures, half of which had been worked on during therapy, comparing naming of these items, with and without the possibility of using the computer prosthesis to generate their own phonemic cues. There were two effects: on both treated and untreated items, patients were better at naming with the prosthesis than without – that is, the benefits of the prosthetic strategy generalized to the untreated items. But there was also a practice effect: in both conditions, items that had been worked on during treatment were named more accurately than those that had not.

Nickels (1992) used a similar strategy in treating patient TRC's naming disorder. TRC was much more accurate at written naming than

Table 4.4: Naming by Bruce and Howard's (1987) patients after learning to use a computer-based aid to generate their own phonemic cues. The benefit from the use of the aid generalizes from treated items to untreated words, but there is also a treatment effect for the treated items in both naming conditions

| | Naming | |
	with aid (%)	without aid (%)
Treated words	57	35
Untreated words	40	29

spoken naming, and benefited from phonemic cues from the therapist. Nickels taught TRC letter-to-sound correspondences, and then to use his knowledge of a word's initial letter to generate his own phonemic cues. As a result of this treatment, TRC's spoken naming (of items not involved in treatment) improved to the level of accuracy of his written naming, and the ability to generate his own cues also benefited his reading aloud to a similar extent.

Table 4.5: Results of Nickels' (1992) treatment of TRC. Development of a self-cueing strategy based on his relatively well-preserved knowledge of written picture names resulted in improvement in both spoken naming and oral reading for items not targeted in treatment

	Pre-therapy (%)	Post-therapy (%)
Spoken naming	8	39
Written naming	49	47
Oral reading	9	38

Both of these examples show generalization. This generalization is found because the treatment enabled the patients to use general strategies to aid spoken word retrieval, and did not directly target the mapping from semantics to phonology.

Cognitive neuropsychology and word retrieval therapy

Because of limitations of space, the evidence discussed above is only a partial account of treatment studies from the CN perspective of the past 15 years (see Nickels and Best, 1996a, 1996b for a more comprehensive review). It is clear, however, that there is accumulating evidence that, even with quite small amounts of treatment, specific treatment techniques can have substantial and long-lasting effects on patients' word retrieval. This evidence comes both from studies of single cases and case series. Cognitive neuropsychology has developed the techniques for studying treatment effects which can show quite conclusively that treatment is effective, using appropriate statistical techniques to analyse the data (see Howard, 1986; Willmes, 1990; Franklin, 1997). As has been pointed out above, many studies of naming therapy show item-specific patterns of improvement. This allows for very simple, but scientifically valid experimental designs. By randomly allocating items to treatment and control conditions (often subject also to matching for initial success rates), and then comparing post-therapy accuracy for the two conditions, it is possible to show that a treatment had a significant, item-specific effect. Thus, it is possible to show that the specified treatment was effective for that subject.

Cognitive neuropsychology has provided the theoretical and practical tools for identifying the level of impairment in word retrieval for a subject. The relationship between levels of breakdown and therapy effects is, however, only beginning to be explored. Is it, for instance, the case that particular types of word retrieval impairment only respond to specific kinds of treatment? Answering this question is not straightforward because of the nature of treatments of word retrieval disorders. If we accept that a spoken or written word will automatically activate both meaning representations and output phonology, then, at an underlying processing level, almost all the treatment techniques are the same, irrespective of whether, on the surface, they emphasize phonological, lexical or semantic processing.

To demonstrate that different types of word retrieval impairment respond only to specific kinds of treatment requires a comparison of different treatments applied to subjects with different levels of impairment. There is some evidence that individual subjects can respond much better to one kind of treatment rather than another (for example, Best et al., 1997; Hillis, 1989; Springer et al., 1991; Nickels and Best, 1996b). Such results, although intriguing, are not necessarily conclusive. This is because a subject might fail to respond to one of the treatments for reasons that are not related directly to the nature of the treatment; they might, for example, fail to practise nearly as much with one treatment (a possibility considered by Best et al., 1997), or the treatment might have happened over a period where, for some reason (feeling a bit ill, depressed, unmotivated ...), the patient was less likely to benefit. This question can only be addressed properly with a prospective case series design where patients with identified levels of impairment are treated with two contrasting therapies. The only study that seems to approach this is the study by Howard et al. (1985b); the evidence, as discussed above, was that patients who benefited from one kind of therapy also improved with the other (although, as I have argued, this may be because the two treatments were very similar in their processing requirements).

When the results of that study are assessed there are seven patients who benefit from treatment and five that do not; this finding is reflected in a statistical result that the treatment effects are non-homogeneous (see also Leach, 1979). Other studies, analysed in this way produce similar findings: for instance, the treatment effects reported by Pring et al. (1993) are also significantly non-homogeneous. Three of the five subjects show substantial and significant treatment effects, and two do not. In neither case is it clear what differentiates the patients who benefit from those who do not.

Single-case studies can only show *after the event* whether or not treatment of a particular type was effective for the patient. A therapist, deciding what treatment strategies to adopt with a particular patient, needs to know *in advance* the probability that a specific treatment strategy will work (see also Howard, 1992). Again this demonstrates a need for prospective case series studies which can examine how different types of patient respond to a treatment – comparing one treatment across subjects. This kind of design can be used to help identify the patient characteristics that determine whether or not a treatment is effective.

The contribution of cognitive neuropsychology to studies of aphasic treatment has been, then, in bringing much greater sophistication to the proper design of the studies and in considering the processes involved in treatment tasks and how this might be effective. A variety of single case and case series studies have shown that specific treatments *can* be effective. The total amount of research work in this area is, still, distressingly limited. We are only beginning to be able to address the important issue of determining which treatment is likely to be most effective for a patient with a particular type of impairment and particular intact processing resources. Answers to these questions are what is really needed to enable therapists to make principled, informed decisions in deciding on the treatment strategy to adopt with an individual patient.

References

Barry C, McHattie J (1991). Depth of semantic processing in picture naming facilitation in aphasic patients. Paper presented at the British Aphasiology Society Conference, Sheffield, September 1991.

Behrmann M, Byng SC (1992). A cognitive approach to the neurorehabilitation of acquired language disorders. In Margolin DI (ed.) Cognitive Neuropsychology in Clinical Practice. New York: Oxford University Press, pp.327–50.

Berman M, Peelle LM (1967). Self-generated cues: a method for aiding aphasic and apractic patients. Journal for Speech and Hearing Disorders 32: 372–6.

Best W, Howard D, Bruce C, Gatehouse C (1997). Cueing the words: a single case study of treatments for anomia. Neuropsychological Rehabilitation 7: 105–41.

Bruce C, Howard D (1987). Computer-generated phonemic cues: an effective aid for naming in aphasia. British Journal of Disorders of Communication 22: 191–201.

Bruce C, Howard D (1988). Why don't Broca's aphasics cue themselves? An investigation of phonemic cueing and tip-of-the-tongue information. Neuropsychologia 26: 253–64.

Caplan D, Vanier M, Baker C (1986). A case study of reproduction conduction aphasia. I: Word production. Cognitive Neuropsychology 3: 99–128.

Caramazza A (1984). The logic of neuropsychological research and the problem of patient classification in aphasia. Brain and Language 21: 9–20.

Caramazza A, Hillis AE (1990). Where do semantic errors come from? Cortex 26: 95–122.

Caramazza A, Hillis AE (1993). For a theory of rehabilitation. Neuropsychological Rehabilitation 3: 217–34.

Coltheart M (1984). Editorial. Cognitive Neuropsychology 1: 1–8.

Coltheart M, Patterson KE, Marshall JC (eds) (1980). Deep Dyslexia. London: Routledge & Kegan Paul.

Coltheart V, Patterson KE, Leahy J (1994). When a ROWS is a ROSE: phonological effects in written word comprehension. Quarterly Journal of Experimental Psychology 47A: 917–55.

de Partz MP (1986). Reeducation of a deep dyslexic patient: rationale of the method and results. Cognitive Neuropsychology 3: 149–77.

Feinberg T, Rothi L, Heilman K (1986). Inner speech in conduction aphasia. Archives of Neurology 43: 591–3.

Franklin SE (1993). Researching the treatment of anomia: the case for single cases. In Stachowiak FJ (ed.) Developments in the Assessment and Rehabilitation of Brain-damaged Patients. Tübingen: Gunter Narr Verlag, pp.273–5.

Franklin SE (1997). Designing single case treatment studies for aphasic patients. Neuropsychological Rehabilitation 7: 401–18.

Frith CD, Friston KJ (1997). Studying brain function with neuroimaging. In Rugg MD (ed.) Cognitive Neuroscience. Hove: Psychology Press, pp.169–95.

Hillis A (1989). Efficacy and generalization of treatment for aphasic naming errors. Archives of Physical Medicine and Rehabilitation 70: 632–6.

Howard D (1986). Beyond randomised controlled trials: the case for effective case studies of the effects of treatment in aphasia. British Journal of Disorders of Communication 21: 89–102.

Howard D (1992). Cognitive neuropsychology and rehabilitation. In von Cramon D, Poeppel E, von Steinbuechel N (eds) Brain Damage and Rehabilitation: A Neuropsychological Approach. Berlin: Springer Verlag, pp.146–54.

Howard D (1997). Language in the human brain. In Rugg MD (ed.) Cognitive Neuroscience. Hove: Psychology Press, pp.277–304.

Howard D, Hatfield FM (1987). Aphasia Therapy; Historical and Contemporary Issues. London: Lawrence Erlbaum.

Howard D, Orchard-Lisle VM (1984). On the origin of semantic errors in naming: evidence from the case of a global aphasic. Cognitive Neuropsychology 1: 163–90.

Howard D, Patterson KE (1992). The Pyramids and Palm Trees Test. Bury St Edmunds: Thames Valley Test Company.

Howard D, Patterson KE, Franklin SE, Orchard-Lisle VM, Morton J (1985a). The facilitation of picture naming in aphasia. Cognitive Neuropsychology 2: 49–80.

Howard D, Patterson KE, Franklin SE, Orchard-Lisle V, Morton J (1985b). The treatment of word retrieval deficits in aphasia: a comparison of two therapy methods. Brain 108: 817–29.

Leach C (1979). Introduction to Statistics: A Non-parametric Approach for the Social Sciences. Chichester: John Wiley.

Le Dorze G, Boulay N, Gaudreau J, Brassard C (1994). The contrasting effects of a semantic versus a fomal-semantic technique for the facilitation of naming in a case of anomia. Aphasiology 8: 127–41.

Levelt WJM (1989). Speaking: From Intention to Articulation. Cambridge, MA: MIT Press.

Levelt WJM, Roelofs A, Meyer AS (1999). A theory of lexical access in speech production. Behavioural and Brain Sciences 22: 1–45.

Marshall J, Pound C, White-Thomson M, Pring TR (1990). The use of picture/word matching tasks to assist word retrieval in aphasic patients. Aphasiology 4: 167–84.

Marshall JC, Newcombe F (1973). Patterns of paralexia; a psycholinguistic approach. Journal for Psycholinguistic Research 2: 175–99.

Miceli G, Amitrano A, Capasso R, Caramazza A (1996). The remediation of anomia resulting from output lexical damage: analysis of two cases. Brain and Language 52: 150–74.

Nickels LA (1992). The autocue? Self-generated phonemic cues in the treatment of a disorder of reading and naming. Cognitive Neuropsychology 9: 155–82.

Nickels LA (1995). Getting it right? Using aphasic naming errors to evaluate theoretical models of spoken word production. Language and Cognitive Processes 10: 13–45.

Nickels LA, Best W (1996a). Therapy for naming disorders (Part I): principles, puzzles and progress. Aphasiology 10: 21–47.

Nickels LA, Best W (1996b). Therapy for naming disorders (Part II): specifics, surprises and suggestions. Aphasiology 10: 109–36.

Nickels LA, Best W (in press). From theory to therapy in aphasia: where are we now and where to next? Neuropsychological Rehabilitation.

Nickels LA, Howard D (1994). A frequent occurrence? Factors affecting the production of semantic errors in aphasic naming. Cognitive Neuropsychology 11: 289–320.

Nickels LA, Howard D (1995). Phonological errors in aphasic naming; comprehension, monitoring and lexicality. Cortex 31: 209–37.

Nickels LA, Howard D (in press). When the words won't come: relating impairments and models of spoken word production. In Wheeldon LR (ed.) Language Production. Hove: Psychology Press.

Patterson KE, Purell C, Morton J (1983). The facilitation of naming in aphasia. In Code C, Muller DJ (eds) Aphasia Therapy. London: Arnold, pp.76–87.

Pease DM, Goodglass H (1978). The effects of cuing on picture naming in aphasia. Cortex 14: 178–89.

Price CJ (1997). The functional anatomy of reading. In Frackowiak RSJ, Friston KJ, Frith CD, Dolan RJ, Mazziotta JC (eds) Human Brain Function. San Diego, CA: Academic Press, pp.301–28.

Pring TR, Davis A, Marshall J (1993). Therapy for word finding deficits: can experimental findings inform clinical work? In Stachowiak FJ (ed.) Developments in the Assessment and Rehabilitation of Brain-damaged Patients. Tübingen: Gunter Narr Verlag, pp.263–71.

Pring T, Hamilton A, Harwood A, Macbride L (1993). Generalization of naming after picture/word matching tasks: only items appearing in therapy benefit. Aphasiology 7: 383–94.

Pring TR, White-Thomson M, Pound C, Marshall J, Davis A (1990). Picture/word matching tasks and word retrieval: some follow-up data and second thoughts. Aphasiology 4: 479–83.

Schriefers H, Meyer AS, Levelt WJM (1990). Exploring the time course of lexical access in language production: picture-word interference studies. Journal of Memory and Language 29: 86–102.

Springer L, Glindemann R, Huber W, Willmes K (1991). How efficacious is PACE-therapy when language systematic training is incorporated? Aphasiology 5: 391–9.

Van Orden GC, Johnston JC, Hale BL (1988). Word identification in reading proceeds from spelling to sound to meaning. Journal of Experimental Psychology: Learning Memory and Cognition 14: 371–86.

Willmes K (1990). Statistical methods for a single-case study approach to aphasia therapy research. Aphasiology 4: 415–36.

Part II
Motor speech disorders

Chapter 5
Dysarthria: clinical features, neuroanatomical framework and assessment

BRUCE E. MURDOCH, ELIZABETH C. WARD and DEBORAH G. THEODOROS

Introduction

Speech production requires the coordinated contraction of a large number of muscles, including the muscles of the lips, jaw, tongue, soft palate, pharynx and larynx as well as the muscles of respiration. Contraction of the muscles of the speech mechanism is, in turn, controlled by nerve impulses that originate in the motor areas of the cerebral cortex and then pass to the muscles by way of the motor pathways, including the descending (upper motor neurone) pathways in the central nervous system and the lower motor neurone pathways distributed by the peripheral nerves (including certain cranial and spinal nerves). Damage to the nervous system causing disruption to any level of the motor system involved in the regulation of the speech mechanism can lead to a disturbance in speech production.

Dysarthria has been defined as 'a collective name for a group of related speech disorders that are due to disturbances in motor control of the speech mechanism resulting from impairment of any of the basic motor processes involved in the execution of speech' (Darley, Aronson and Brown, 1975: 2). According to this definition, the term 'dysarthria' should be applied only to those speech disorders that result from damage to the central or peripheral nervous system (that is, those speech disorders that have a neurogenic origin) and should not be applied to those speech disorders associated with either somatic structural defects (for example, cleft palate, congenitally enlarged pharynx, congenitally short palate and malocclusion) or psychosocial disorders (for example, psychogenic aphonia).

Depending on which level(s) of the motor system is affected, a number of different types of dysarthria may be recognized, each of which is characterized by its own set of auditory perceptual features.

Over the years, a variety of different systems have been used to classify the various types of dysarthria (for example, age at onset (congenital and acquired dysarthria); neurological diagnosis (vascular dysarthria, neoplastic dysarthria and so on); site of lesion (cerebellar dysarthria, lower motor neurone dysarthria and so on)). The system of classification most universally accepted by speech pathologists and neurologists, however, and therefore the system most used clinically is the perceptually based classification scheme devised by Darley et al. (1975). The six types of dysarthria identified by the Darley et al. (1975) system, together with their localization, are listed in Table 5.1.

Table 5.1: Clinically recognized types of dysarthria together with their lesion sites

Dysarthria type	Lesion site
Flaccid dysarthria	Lower motor neurones
Spastic dysarthria	Upper motor neurones
Hypokinetic dysarthria	Basal ganglia and associated brainstem nuclei
Hyperkinetic dysarthria	Basal ganglia and associated brainstem nuclei
Ataxic dysarthria	Cerebellum and/or its connections
Mixed dysarthria	
for example, mixed flaccid-spastic dysarthria	Both lower and upper motor neurones (for example, amyotrophic lateral sclerosis)
mixed ataxic-spastic-flaccid dysarthria	Cerebellum/cerebellar connections, upper motor neurones and lower motor neurones (for example, Wilson's disease)

Each of these different types of dysarthria is described below in terms of their neuroanatomical framework and clinical features, including their perceptual, acoustic and physiological characteristics.

Flaccid dysarthria

Neuroanatomical framework of flaccid dysarthria

Flaccid dysarthria is a collective name for the group of speech disorders arising from damage to either the lower motor neurones supplying the muscles of the speech mechanism and/or the muscles of the speech mechanism themselves. The term flaccid dysarthria is derived from the major symptom of lower motor neurone damage, namely flaccid paralysis. Lower motor neurones form the ultimate pathway (that is, the final common pathway) through which nerve impulses are conveyed from the central nervous system to the skeletal muscles, including the muscles of the speech mechanism. The cell bodies of the lower motor neurones are located in either the motor nuclei of the cranial nerves or in the anterior horns of the spinal cord. From this location, the axons of the lower motor neurones pass via the various motor cranial nerves and spinal nerves of the peripheral nervous system to the skeletal muscles. Lesions of the motor cranial nerves and spinal nerves represent lower motor neurone lesions and interrupt the conduction of nerve impulses from the central nervous system to the muscles. Consequently, voluntary control of the affected muscles is lost. Simultaneously, in that the nerve impulses necessary for the maintenance of muscle tone are also lost, the muscles involved become flaccid (hypotonic). Muscle weakness, a loss or reduction of muscle reflexes, atrophy of the muscles involved and fasciculation (spontaneous twitches of individual muscle bundles – fascicles) are further characteristics of lower motor neurone lesions. All or some of these characteristics may be manifest in the muscles of the speech mechanisms of persons with flaccid dysarthria, with hypotonia, weakness and reduced reflex activity representing the primary characteristics of flaccid paralysis. The actual lower motor neurones, which, if damaged, may be associated with flaccid dysarthria, are listed in Table 5.2.

Table 5.2: Lower motor neurones associated with flaccid dysarthria

Speech process	Muscle	Site of cell body	Nerves through which axons pass
Respiration	Diaphragm	3rd-5th cervical segments of spinal cord	Phrenic nerves
Phonation	Laryngeal muscles	Nucleus ambiguus in medulla oblongata	Vagus nerves (X)
Articulation	Pterygoids, masseter, temporalis, etc.	Motor nucleus of trigeminal in pons	Trigeminal nerves (V)
	Facial expression, for example, orbicularis oris	Facial nucleus in pons	Facial nerves (VII)
	Tongue muscles	Hypoglossal nucleus in medulla oblongata	Hypoglossal nerves (XII)
Resonation	Levator veli palatini	Nucleus ambiguus in medulla oblongata	Vagus nerves (X)
	Tensor veli palatini	Motor nucleus of trigeminal in pons	Trigeminal nerves (V)

Neurological disorders associated with flaccid dysarthria

With the exception of the muscles of respiration, the motor cranial nerves which arise from the bulbar region (pons and medulla oblongata) of the brainstem (that is, cranial nerves V, VII, IX, X, XI and XII) innervate the muscles of the speech mechanism. Bulbar palsy, the name commonly given to flaccid paralysis of the muscles supplied by the cranial nerves arising from the bulbar region of the brainstem, can be caused by a variety of conditions which may either affect the cell body of the lower motor neurones or the axons of the lower motor neurones as they course through the peripheral nerves. The major disorders of lower motor neurones which can cause flaccid dysarthria are listed in Table 5.3.

Table 5.3: Neurological disorders associated with flaccid dysarthria

Site of lesion	Disorder	Aetiology	Signs and symptoms
A. Peripheral nerves (especially cranial nerves V, VII, IX, X, XI and XII).	Polyneuritis	Inflammation of a number of nerves. Acute type – may follow viral infections, for example, glandular fever Chronic type – may be associated with diabetes mellitus and alcohol abuse.	Sensory and lower motor neurone changes usually begin in the distal portion of the limbs and spread to involve other regions including the face, tongue, soft palate, pharynx and larynx. The muscles of respiration may also be involved. Bilateral facial paralysis may occur in idiopathic polyneuritis (Guillain-Barr (syndrome).
	Compression of and damage to cranial nerves	Neoplasm, for example, acoustic neuroma, causing compression of the VIIth nerve. Aneurysm, for example, compression of the left recurrent layngeal nerve by an aortic arch aneurysm Trauma, for example, damage to the recurrent laryngeal nerve during thyroidectomy	Localized lower motor neurone signs dependent on the particular nerves involved.
	Idiopathic facial paralysis (Bell's palsy)	Pathogenesis unknown in most cases but may be related to inflammatory lesions in the stylomastoid foramen. Approximately 80% of cases recover.	Abrupt onset of unilateral facial paralysis.

Table 5.3: (contd)

Site of lesion	Disorder	Aetiology	Signs and symptoms
B. Cranial nerve nuclei and/or anterior horns of spinal cord	Brainstem cerebrovascular accidents	Lateral medullary syndrome (Wallenberg's syndrome) – caused by occlusion of the posterior-interior cerebellar artery, vertebral artery or lateral medullary artery.	Damage to the nucleus ambiguus (origin of the IXth, Xth and cranial portion of the XIth nerve) leads to dysphagia, hoarseness and paralysis of the soft palate on the side of the lesion. Impaired sensation over the face, vertigo and nausea are also present.
		Medial medullary syndrome - caused by occlusion of the anterior spinal or vertebral arteries.	Damage to the hypoglossal nucleus leads to unilateral paralysis and atrophy of the tongue. A crossed hemiparesis (sparing the face) and sensory changes are also present.
		Lateral pontine syndrome (Foville's syndrome) – caused by occlusion of the anterior-interior cerebellar artery or circumferential artery.	Damage to the facial nucleus causes flaccid paralysis of the facial muscles on the side of the lesion. Other symptoms may include deafness, ataxic gait, vertigo, nausea and sensory changes.
		Medial pontine syndrome (Millard-Gubler syndrome) – caused by occlusion of the paramedian branch of the basilar artery.	Symptoms include facial paralysis on the side of lesion, diplopia, crossed hemiparesis and impaired touch and position sense.
	Progressive bulbar palsy	A type of motor neurone disease in which there is progressive degeneration of the motor cells in some cranial nerve nuclei.	Progressive weakness and atrophy of the muscles of the speech mechanism.
	Poliomyelitis	Viral infection which affects the motor nuclei of the cranial nerves and the anterior horn cells of the spinal cord.	Paralysis and wasting of affected muscles with lower motor neurone signs. Paralysis may be widespread or localized and can affect the speech muscles, limb muscles and muscles of respiration.

(contd)

Table 5.3: (contd)

Site of lesion	Disorder	Aetiology	Signs and symptoms
	Neoplasm	Brainstem tumours – these are more common in children than adult.	Tumour may progressively involve the cranial nerve nuclei causing gradual weakness and flaccid paralysis of the muscles of the speech mechanism.
	Syringobulbia	Slowly progressive cystic degeneration in the lower brainstem in the region of the 4th ventricle. Congenital disorder with onset of symptoms usually in early adult life.	As the cystic cavity develops there may be progressive involvement of the cranial nerve nuclei leading to lower motor neurone signs in the muscles of the speech mechanism.
	Mobius syndrome (congenital facial diplegia)	Congenital hyperplasia of the VIth and VIIth cranial nerve nuclei	Bilateral facial palsy (VII) and bilateral abducens palsy (VI)

Flaccid dysarthria can also be caused by conditions that either impair nerve impulse transmission across the neuromuscular junction (for example, myasthenia gravis, Eaton-Lambert syndrome, botulinum toxin) or disorders that involve the muscles of the speech mechanism directly (for example, muscular dystrophy, polymyositis).

Clinical characteristics of flaccid dysarthria

The specific characteristics of the speech disorder manifest in patients with flaccid dysarthria varies from case to case, depending on which particular nerves are affected and the relative degree of weakness resulting from the damage. A number of subtypes of flaccid dysarthria are therefore recognized, each with their own speech characteristics determined by the specific nerve or combination of nerves involved.

(a) Trigeminal, facial and hypoglossal nerve lesions

The functioning of the articulators (that is, tongue, lips, jaw and so on) is regulated by the Vth (trigeminal), VIIth (facial) and XIIth (hypoglossal) nerves. The trigeminal nerves are the largest of the cranial nerves and emerge from the brainstem on the lateral sides of the pons. Each trigeminal nerve divides into three branches, the ophthalmic branch, the maxillary branch and the mandibular branch. Both the ophthalmic and maxillary branches are purely sensory, whereas the mandibular branch is mixed sensory and motor: consequently, it is the mandibular branch which, if damaged, can cause flaccid dysarthria. The motor fibres of the mandibular branch innervate the muscles of mastication, which include the temporalis, masseter and medial and lateral pterygoid muscles. In addition, the motor fibres also supply the mylohyoid, anterior belly of the digastric, the tensor veli palatini and the tensor tympani of the middle ear.

Bilateral trigeminal lesions may leave the elevators of the mandible (for example, the masseter and temporalis muscles) too weak to approximate the mandible and maxilla. This, in turn, may prevent the tongue and lips from making the contacts with oral structures required for the production of labial and lingual consonants and vowels, with devastating consequences for speech intelligibility. In contrast, unilateral trigeminal lesions cause only a minor impairment to the patient's ability to elevate their mandible and consequently are associated with only a minor effect on speech intelligibility. In most cases, lesions to the trigeminal nerves usually occur in combination with lesions to other cranial nerves, isolated trigeminal lesions occurring only rarely.

The facial nerves emerge from the lateral aspects of the brainstem at the lower border of the pons, in the ponto-medullary sulcus, in the form of two distinct bundles of fibres of unequal size. The larger, more medial bundle arises from the facial nucleus of the pons and carries motor fibres to the muscles of facial expression, including the occipito-frontalis, orbicularis oris and buccinator. Other muscles supplied by the facial nerves include the stylohyoid, the posterior belly of the digastric and the stapedius in the middle ear. The smaller bundle carries autonomic fibres and is known as the nervus intermedius. Lesions in one or other of the facial nerves lead to unilateral flaccid paralysis on the ipsilateral side of the face, causing distortion of bilabial and labio-dental consonants. Because of the weakness of the lips on the affected side, patients with unilateral facial paralysis are unable to seal their lips sufficiently to prevent air escaping from the mouth during the build-up of intra-oral pressure. Consequently, the production of plosives, in particular, is defective. These symptoms are more extreme in patients with bilateral facial paralysis (for example, as occurs in Mobius syndrome), the bilateral weakness leading to speech impairments ranging from distortion to complete obliteration of bilabial and labio-dental consonants. Vowel distortion may also be evident in severe cases owing to problems with either lip rounding or lip spreading. Lesions involving the VIIth nerves can occur in isolation or in combination with other cranial nerves.

Each hypoglossal nerve emerges from the medulla oblongata as a series of rootlets in the groove that separates the pyramid and olive. The hypoglossal nerves innervate all of the intrinsic and most of the extrinsic tongue muscles, with the exception of the palatoglossus. Other muscles in the region of the neck also supplied by the hypoglossal nerves include the sternohyoid, the sternothyroid, the inferior belly of the omohyoid and the geniohyoid muscles. By interfering with normal tongue movements, lesions of the hypoglossal nerves cause disturbances in articulation. Unilateral hypoglossal lesions cause ipsilateral paralysis of the tongue and may result from either brainstem conditions such as medial medullary syndrome or peripheral nerve lesions such as submaxillary tumours compressing one or other of the hypoglossal nerves. Although this may be associated with mild, temporary articulatory imprecision, especially during production of linguo-dental and linguo-palatal consonants, in most cases the patient learns to compensate rapidly for the unilateral tongue weakness or paralysis. Bilateral hypoglossal lesions, however, are associated with more severe articulatory disturbances. In such cases, tongue movement may be severely restricted and speech sounds such as high front vowels and consonants that require elevation of the tip of the tongue to the upper alveolar ridge or hard palate (for example, /t/, /d/, /n/, /l/ and so on) may be grossly distorted.

(b) Vagus nerve lesions

Each vagus nerve arises from the lateral surface of the medulla oblongata as a series of rootlets which lie in the post-olivary sulcus immediately inferior to those that give rise to the glossopharyngeal nerve. The vagus nerves each contain sensory, motor and autonomic fibres. The motor fibres of the vagus arise from the nucleus ambiguus, with additional motor fibres joining the vagus from the cranial portion of the XIth (accessory) nerve. In combination, the motor fibres supply the muscles of the pharynx, larynx and the levator veli palatini and musculus uvulae of the soft palate. The first branch of the vagus nerve important for speech is the pharyngeal nerve, which supplies the levator muscles of the soft palate. As the vagus descends in the neck it gives off a second branch, the superior laryngeal nerve, which supplies the crico-thyroid muscle (the chief tensor muscle of the vocal cords). At a lower level in the neck a third branch is given off, the recurrent laryngeal nerve, which supplies all of the intrinsic muscles of the larynx except for the crico-thyroid and is, therefore, responsible for regulating adduction of the vocal cords for phonation, and abduction of the vocal cords for unvoiced phonemes and inspiration.

Lesions that involve the nucleus ambiguus in the brainstem (intramedullary lesions) (as occurs in lateral medullary syndrome) or the vagus nerve near to the brainstem (extramedullary lesions) (for example, in the region of the jugular foramen) cause paralysis of all muscles that are supplied by the vagus. In such cases, the vocal cord on the affected side is paralysed in a slightly abducted position, leading to flaccid dysphonia characterized by moderate breathiness, harshness and reduced volume. Additional voice characteristics that may also be present include diplophonia, short phrases and inhalatory stridor. The soft palate on the same side is also paralysed, causing hypernasality in the patient's speech. If the lesion is bilateral, the vocal cords on both sides are paralysed and can be neither abducted nor adducted and elevation of the soft palate is also impaired bilaterally, causing more severe breathiness and hypernasality. The major clinical signs of bilateral flaccid vocal cord paralysis include breathy voice (reflecting incomplete adduction of the vocal cords that results in excessive air escape), audible inhalation (inspiratory stridor – reflecting inadequate abduction of the vocal cords during inspiration), and abnormally short phrases during contextual speech (possibly as a consequence of excessive air loss during speech as a result of inefficient laryngeal valving). Other signs seen in some patients include monotony of pitch and monotony of loudness. Bilateral weakness of the soft palate is associated with hypernasality, audible nasal emission, reduced sharpness of consonant production (as a consequence of reduced intraoral pressure due to nasal escape) and short phrases (reflecting premature exhaustion of expiratory air supply as a result of nasal escape).

Lesions to the vagus nerve distal to the branch that supplies the soft palate (the pharyngeal branch) but proximal to the exit of the superior laryngeal nerve have the same effect on phonation as brainstem lesions. However, such lesions do not produce hypernasality since functioning of the levator veli palatini is not compromised. Lesions limited to the recurrent laryngeal nerves (as may occur as a consequence of damage during thyroidectomy or as a result of compression of the vagus by intra-thoracic masses or aortic arch aneurysms) are also associated with dysphonia. In this latter case, however, the crico-thyroid muscles (the principal tensor muscles of the vocal cords) are not affected and the vocal cords are paralysed closer to the midline (the para-median position). Consequently, the voice is likely to be harsh and reduced in loudness, but with a lesser degree of breathiness than seen in cases with brainstem lesions involving the nucleus ambiguus. Bilateral damage to the recurrent laryngeal nerves is rare. If present, bilateral paralysis of the vocal cords is more likely to have resulted from a brainstem lesion.

(c) Phrenic and intercostal nerve lesions

The muscles of respiration are important for the motor production of speech in that the exhaled breath provides the power source for speech. It follows, therefore, that interruption of the nerve supply to the respiratory muscles would interfere with normal speech production.

Lesions involving either the phrenic or intercostal nerves may lead to respiratory hypofunction in the form of a reduced tidal volume and vital capacity and impaired control of expiration. In general, diffuse impairment of the intercostal nerves is required to have any major effect on respiration. Spinal injuries that damage the 3rd to 5th segments of the cervical spinal cord (that is, the origin of the phrenic nerves) can paralyse the diaphragm bilaterally, thereby leading to significant impairment of respiration. Respiratory hypofunction may in turn affect the patient's speech, resulting in speech abnormalities such as short phrases owing to more rapid exhaustion of breath during speech and possibly to a reduction in pitch and loudness as a result of limited expiratory flow volume.

(d) Multiple cranial nerve lesions

Multiple cranial nerve lesions are most commonly caused by intracranial conditions affecting the brainstem. In that the functioning of several cranial nerves is compromised simultaneously, the resulting flaccid dysarthria is usually severe. For example, in bulbar palsy the muscles supplied by cranial nerves V, VII, IX, X, XI and XII may dysfunction simultaneously. As a result, functioning of the muscles of the lips, tongue, jaw, palate and larynx are affected in varying combinations and with varying degrees of weakness. Disorders evident in the affected person's speech may include hypernasality with nasal emission owing to disruption of the palatopharyngeal valve; breathiness, harsh voice, audible inspiration, monopitch and monoloudness associated with laryngeal dysfunction; and distortion of consonant production owing to impairment of the articulators.

(e) Myasthenia gravis

Myasthenia gravis is a condition characterized by muscle weakness that progressively worsens as the muscle is used (fatigability) and rapidly recovers when the muscle is at rest. The condition represents a disorder of neuromuscular transmission possibly caused by an autoimmune attack on the acetylcholine receptors on the muscle fibres. This, in turn, causes the muscle to become less responsive to the acetylcholine that triggers its contraction.

For a long time the abnormal muscular fatigability may be confined to, or predominate in, an isolated group of muscles. For instance, ptosis of one or both upper eyelids caused by weakness of the levator palpebrae is often one of the first symptoms of the condition. Facial, jaw, bulbar and neck muscle weakness ultimately develops in about 50% of cases. As these patients speak, fatigue of the muscles supplied by the bulbar cranial nerves becomes more and more evident, resulting in increasing levels of hypernasality, deterioration of articulation, onset and increase of dysphonia and a reduction in loudness levels. Eventually speech becomes unintelligible.

Spastic dysarthria

The term 'spastic dysarthria' was used by Darley et al. (1975) to describe the speech disturbance seen in association with damage to the upper motor neurones (that is, the neurones that convey nerve impulses from the motor areas of the cerebral cortex to the lower motor neurones). The system of classification devised by Darley et al. (1975) was based on classifying the neuromuscular status of the muscles whose dysfunction caused the dysarthria. The reference to 'spastic' in the term 'spastic dysarthria' is, therefore, a reflection of the clinical signs of upper motor neurone damage present in the bulbar musculature of these patients, which include spastic paralysis or paresis of the involved muscles; hyper-reflexia (for example, hyperactive jaw-jerk); little or no muscle atrophy; and the presence of pathological reflexes (for example, sucking reflex).

Neuroanatomical framework of spastic dysarthria

Lesions that disrupt the upper motor neurones causing spastic dysarthria can be located in the cerebral cortex, the internal capsule, the cerebral peduncles or the brainstem. The upper motor neurone system can be divided into two major components, one a direct component and the other an indirect component. In the direct component the axons of the upper motor neurones descend from their cell bodies in the motor cortex to the level of the lower motor neurones without interruption (that is, without synapsing). The direct component is also known as the pyramidal system. The indirect component, previously called the extrapyramidal system, descends to the level of the lower motor neurone by way of a multi-synaptic pathway involving structures such as the basal ganglia, thalamus, reticular formation and so on, on the way. The indirect motor system appears to be primarily responsible for postural arrangements and the orientation of movement in space, whereas the pyramidal system is chiefly responsible for controlling the far more discrete and skilled voluntary aspects of a movement. Because in most locations (for example, the internal capsule) the two systems lie in close anatomical proximity, lesions that affect one component will usually also involve the other component. The term 'upper motor neurone lesion' is usually not applied to disorders affecting only the extrapyramidal system (for example, in basal ganglia lesions). Such disorders are termed 'extrapyramidal syndromes' and include conditions such as Parkinson's syndrome, chorea, athetosis and so on, which are discussed under hypokinetic and hyperkinetic dysarthria below.

The pyramidal system can be subdivided into those fibres that project to the spinal cord and those that project to the brainstem. In all, three major fibre groups comprise the pyramidal system; the cortico-spinal tracts (pyramidal system proper); the cortico-mesencephalic tracts; and the cortico-bulbar tracts. The cortico-spinal tracts descend from the cerebral cortex via the internal capsule and pyramids to various levels of the spinal cord where they synapse with lower motor neurones. Near to the junction of the medulla oblongata and the spinal cord, the majority (85–90%) of the fibres in each pyramid cross to the opposite side, interlacing as they do so and forming the decussation of the pyramids. It is this crossing that provides the contralateral motor control of the limbs, the motor cortex controlling movement of the right limbs and vice versa.

The cortico-mesencephalic tracts are composed of fibres that descend from the cerebral cortex to the nuclei of cranial nerves III, IV and VI, which provide the motor supply to the extrinsic muscles of the eye. The fibres arise from the frontal eye field, which is that part of the cerebral cortex of the frontal lobe that lies immediately anterior to the pre-motor cortex.

The fibres of the cortico-bulbar tracts start out in company with those of the cortico-spinal tracts but take a divergent route at the level of the mid-brain. They terminate by synapsing with lower motor neurones in the nuclei of cranial nerves V, VII, IX, X, XI and XII. For this reason, they form the most important component of the pyramidal system in relation to the occurrence of spastic dysarthria. Although the majority of cortico-bulbar fibres cross to the contralateral side, uncrossed (ipsilateral) connections also exist. In fact, most of the motor nuclei of the cranial nerves in the brainstem receive bilateral upper motor neurone connections. Consequently, although to a varying degree the predominance of upper motor neurone innervation to the cranial nerve nuclei comes from the contralateral hemisphere, in most instances there is also considerable ipsilateral upper motor neurone innervation. One important exception to the above upper motor neurone innervation of the cranial nerve nuclei is that part of the facial nucleus that gives rise to the lower motor neurones that supply the lower half of the face. It seems to receive only a contralateral upper motor neurone connection.

Clinically, the presence of a bilateral innervation to most cranial nerve nuclei has important implications for the type of speech disorder that follows unilateral upper motor neurone lesions. Although a mild and usually transient impairment in articulation may occur subsequent to unilateral cortico-bulbar lesions, in general bilateral cortico-bulbar lesions are required to produce a permanent dysarthria.

Unilateral upper motor neurone lesions located in either the motor cortex or internal capsule cause a spastic paralysis or weakness in the contralateral lower half of the face, but not the upper part of the face which may be associated with a mild, transient dysarthria due to weakness of orbicularis oris. There is no weakness of the forehead, muscles of mastication, soft palate (that is, no hypernasality), pharynx (that is, no swallowing problems) or larynx (that is, no dysphonia). A unilateral upper motor neurone lesion may, however, produce a mild unilateral weakness of the tongue on the side opposite the lesion. In the case of such a unilateral lesion it seems, therefore, that the ipsilateral upper motor neurone is adequate to maintain near-normal function of most bulbar muscles, except those in the tongue. Although most authors agree that the hypoglossal nucleus receives bilateral upper motor neurone innervation, for some reason the ipsilateral connection seems to be less effective than in the case of other cranial nerve nuclei.

Neurological disorders associated with spastic dysarthria

Damage to the upper motor neurones is associated with two major syndromes: Pseudobulbar palsy (also called supranuclear bulbar palsy) and spastic hemiplegia. Both of these conditions are characterized by spasticity and impairment or loss of voluntary movements.

Pseudobulbar palsy takes its name from its clinical resemblance to bulbar palsy (pseudo='false') and is associated with a variety of neurological disorders which bilaterally disrupt the upper motor neurone connections to the bulbar cranial nerves (for example, bilateral cerebrovascular accidents, traumatic brain injury, extensive brain tumours, degenerative neurological conditions such as motor neurone disease). In this condition, the bulbar muscles, including the muscles of articulation, the velopharynx and larynx are hypertonic and exhibit hyper-reflexia. In addition, there is a reduction in the range and force of movement of the bulbar muscles as well as slowness of individual and repetitive movements. The rhythm of repetitive movements, however, is regular and the direction of movement normal. Symptoms of pseudobulbar palsy include bilateral facial paralysis, dysarthria, dysphonia, bilateral hemiparesis, incontinence and bradykinesia. Drooling from the corners of the mouth is common and many of these patients exhibit lability. A hyperactive jaw reflex and positive sucking reflex are also evident and swallowing problems are a common feature.

In contrast, unilateral upper motor neurone lesions produce spastic hemiplegia, a condition in which the muscles of the lower face and extremities on the opposite side of the body are primarily affected. The bulbar muscles are not greatly affected, with weakness being confined to the contralateral lips, lower half of the face and tongue. In addition, the forehead, palate, pharynx and larynx are largely unaffected. Consequently, unlike pseudobulbar palsy, spastic hemiplegia is not associated with problems in mastication, swallowing, velopharyngeal function or laryngeal activity. The tongue appears normal in the mouth but deviates to the weaker side on protrusion. Only a transitory dysarthria comprising a mild articulatory imprecision rather than a persistent spastic dysarthria is present.

Clinical characteristics of spastic dysarthria

All aspects of speech production including articulation, resonance, phonation and respiration are affected in spastic dysarthria but to varying degrees. The condition is characterized by slow and laboured speech which is produced only with considerable effort. Based on the findings of a perceptual analysis, Darley, Aronson and Brown (1969a, b) found that the deviant speech characteristics of spastic dysarthria clustered primarily in the areas of articulatory incompetence, phonatory stenosis and prosodic insufficiency.

Darley et al. (1969a) identified the most predominant perceptual features of spastic dysarthria as: imprecise consonants, monopitch, reduced stress, harsh voice quality, monoloudness, low pitch, slow rate, hypernasality, strained strangled voice quality, short phrases, distorted vowels, pitch breaks, continuous breathy voice, and excess and equal stress. Chenery, Murdoch and Ingram (1992) identified a similar set of deviant perceptual features in their group of subjects with pseudobulbar palsy, thereby confirming that subjects with spastic dysarthria present with deficits in all aspects of speech production (that is, respiration, phonation, resonation, articulation and prosody). A similar profile of deviant speech dimensions was reported by Thompson and Murdoch (1995a) in a group of non-pseudobulbar palsy subjects with mild to moderate spastic dysarthria subsequent to cerebrovascular accident.

To date, very few instrumental investigations have been conducted to examine the physiological impairments underlying the deviant perceptual speech dimensions observed in patients with spastic dysarthria. Consequently, there is still a need for further research into the nature and type of physiological deficits occurring in the speech mechanism of persons in this group. In general, the findings of those physiological and acoustic studies that have been reported tend to support the results of the perceptual investigations, indicating the presence of deficits in the function of all aspects of the speech production mechanism in persons with spastic dysarthria.

Respiratory function in spastic dysarthria

Murdoch, Noble, Chenery and Ingram (1989) investigated the respiratory function of five subjects with pseudobulbar palsy using both spirometric and kinematic assessments. Of their subject group, four of the five subjects exhibited reduced vital capacities on standard spirometric assessments. The kinematic assessment of the dysarthric group revealed irregularities in the chest wall movements of the diaphragm and abdomen which occurred during vowel and syllable production tasks but not during reading tasks (Murdoch et al., 1989). Volume excursions during reading and conversation tasks were also found to be reduced.

On the basis of these findings, it was concluded that the identified respiratory impairments had the potential to interfere with speech production, particularly where speech is associated with respiratory effort above normal tidal volume (Murdoch et al., 1989).

In a more recent study (Thompson, 1995), the respiratory function and speech breathing abilities of a group of 18 subjects with mild to moderate spastic dysarthria following cerebrovascular accident (CVA) were investigated. In contrast to the results of Murdoch et al. (1989), the results of the kinematic assessments conducted by Thompson (1995) revealed that the dysarthric subjects had normal respiratory parameters during reading and conversational speech tasks. Analysis of the kinematic patterns during the production of the maximum effort speech tasks, however, identified reduced lung volumes in the CVA group, consistent with the Murdoch et al. (1989) study. Particularly during the production of maximum effort tasks there was evidence to suggest that the reduced lung volumes observed in the CVA group were contributed to by reduced ribcage and abdominal expansion during inspiration as well as reduced abdominal contraction during expiration, possibly as a result of the presence of spasticity or weakness of the chest wall muscles. Spirometric analysis also confirmed reduced lung volumes and capacities in the dysarthric subject group (Thompson, 1995).

Laryngeal function in spastic dysarthria

Since Darley et al. (1969a, b) described the primary vocal qualities of spastic dysarthria as 'strained-strangled' and 'harsh', it has been presumed that the neurological damage to the upper motor neurones of these subjects results in hyperadduction of the laryngeal muscles and surrounding supraglottic musculature, leading to a narrowing of the laryngeal aperture.

Given the speculated presence of laryngeal hyperadduction, it would be expected that physiological investigations of laryngeal function of subjects with spastic dysarthria would reveal behaviours characteristic of laryngeal hyperfunction. The results of a recent investigation (Murdoch, Thompson and Stokes, 1994) into the laryngeal function of subjects with predominantly mild to moderate spastic dysarthria following CVA, however, only partly confirmed the presence of hyperfunctional laryngeal parameters in subjects with spastic dysarthria. Using both electroglottographic and aerodynamic techniques, Murdoch et al. (1994) found that only 50% of their group of dysarthric subjects exhibited a predominance of features classically associated with hyperfunctional laryngeal activity, including increased resistance, elevated pressures and decreased laryngeal airflow. Even then, not all of these features were always evident in the same subject, with the results of a cluster analysis identifying three different subgroups with varying combinations of hyperfunctional features. The remaining 50% of the CVA subjects in the Murdoch et al. (1994) investigation were collected into a single 'hypofunctional' subgroup, their performance on the instrumental measures demonstrating lower than normal resistance and higher than normal airflow during phonation, features more frequently associated with laryngeal hypofunction. Replication of this investigation including subjects with more severe degrees of spastic dysarthria, and incorporating a direct examination of laryngeal behaviour and electromyographic recordings of vocal muscle tone would provide greater insight into the laryngeal behaviours of this subject group.

Articulatory function in spastic dysarthria

Deficits in articulatory function, particularly reduced movement of the lips and tongue (Enderby, 1986), have been identified as a characteristic feature of subjects with spastic dysarthria. Instrumental studies have also confirmed a reduced range of articulatory movement and a slowing down in the rate of speech in patients with spastic dysarthria (Hirose, Kiritani and Sawashima, 1980, 1982b; Ziegler and Von Cramon, 1986), together with a reduction in maximum tongue pressures (Thompson, Murdoch and Stokes 1995a). Impairments in maximum force repetition rate and endurance capabilities have also been reported in the labial function of subjects with upper motor neurone damage (Thompson, Murdoch and Stokes, 1995b).

Velopharyngeal function in spastic dysarthria

Hypernasality is a commonly reported feature of spastic dysarthria. Thompson and Murdoch (1995b) investigated the presence of nasality disturbances in a group of 18 dysarthric subjects with upper motor neurone damage following CVA. They used the accelerometric assessment technique to indirectly evaluate the functioning of the velopharyngeal component of the speech mechanism in these subjects. The results of their investigation revealed that the CVA subjects as a group, produced a significantly higher degree of nasality on the production of non-nasal speech tasks than the control subjects. The results of the individual evaluation of each subject, however, revealed that less than half of the subjects presented with disorders of nasal resonance, indicating a relatively low incidence of nasality disorders in subjects with predominantly mild and mild-moderate degrees of spastic dysarthria. No subject was found to have hyponasality on the basis of the instrumental assessment.

The presence of hypernasality in the speech of subjects with spastic dysarthria has been attributed to the presence of slow and incomplete elevation of the soft palate (Chenery et al., 1992). Based on personal observations made during cineradiography, Aten (1983) reported that, following initial elevation, there is progressive failure of velar closure in spastic dysarthric patients when counting or during production of serial speech. In subjects with more severe resonance disorders, Aten (1983) describes an 'inertia in initiating speech activities' (p.70) which is not actually weakness but rather 'a rapid onset of increased resistance to stretch' (p.70) which blocks the normal movement of the velum (Aten, 1983).

Ataxic dysarthria

Damage to the cerebellum or its connections leads to a condition called 'ataxia', in which movements become uncoordinated. If the ataxia affects the muscles of the speech mechanism, the production of speech may become abnormal, leading to a cluster of deviant speech dimensions collectively referred to as 'ataxic dysarthria'.

Although even simple movements are affected by cerebellar damage, the movements most disrupted by cerebellar disorders are the more complex, multi-component sequential movements. Following damage to the cerebellum, complex movements tend to be broken down or decomposed into their individual sequential components, each of which may be executed with errors of force, amplitude and timing, leading to uncoordinated movements. As speech production requires the coordinated and simultaneous contraction of a large number of muscle groups, it is easy to understand how cerebellar disorders could disrupt speech production and cause ataxic dysarthria. To fully understand the pathophysiological basis of ataxic dysarthria, however, requires an understanding of the basic neuroanatomy and functional neurology of the cerebellum.

Neuroanatomical framework of ataxic dysarthria

Located in the posterior cranial fossa, the cerebellum is composed of two large cerebellar hemispheres connected by a mid-portion called the vermis. As in the case of the cerebral hemispheres, the cerebellar hemispheres are covered by a layer of grey matter or cortex. Unlike the cerebral cortex, however, the cerebellar cortex is uniform in structure throughout its extent. The cerebellar cortex is highly folded into thin transverse folds or folia. A series of deep and definite fissures divide the cerebellum into a number of lobes. Most authors recognize the presence of three lobes: the anterior lobe, the posterior lobe and the flocculonodular lobe. The posterior lobe, also referred to as the neocerebellum, is the largest of the three lobes and is the most concerned with regulation of voluntary muscle activities. It has an essential role in the coordination of phasic movements and consequently is the most important part of the cerebellum for the coordination of speech movements.

The central core of the cerebellum, like that of the cerebral hemispheres, is made up of white matter. Located within the white matter, on either side of the midline, are four grey masses, called the cerebellar or deep nuclei. These are composed of the dentate nucleus, the globose and emboliform nuclei (collectively referred to as the interpositus) and the fastigial nucleus. The majority of Purkinje cell axons, which carry impulses away from the cerebellar cortex, terminate in these nuclei.

Although the cerebellum does not, itself, initiate any muscle contractions, it monitors those areas of the brain that do in order to coordinate the actions of muscle groups and time their contractions so that movements involving the skeletal muscles are performed smoothly and accurately. It is thought that the cerebellum achieves this coordination by translating the motor intent of the individual into response parameters that then control the action of the peripheral muscles. In order to be able to perform its primary function of synergistic coordination of muscular activity, the cerebellum requires extensive connections with other parts of the nervous system. Damage to the pathways comprising these connections can cause cerebellar dysfunction and possible ataxic dysarthria, the same as damage to the cerebellum itself. Briefly, the cerebellum functions in part by comparing input from the motor cortex with information concerning the momentary status of muscle contraction, degree of tension of the muscle tendons, position of parts of the body and forces acting on the surfaces of the body originating from muscle spindles, Golgi tendon organs and so on, and then sending appropriate messages back to the motor cortex to ensure smooth, coordinated muscle function. Consequently, the cerebellum requires input from the motor cortex, from muscle and joint receptors, receptors in the internal ear detecting changes in the position and rate of rotation of the head, skin receptors and so on. Conversely, pathways carrying signals from the cerebellum back to the cortex are also required.

Connections with other parts of the brain are provided on either side by three bundles of nerve fibres called the cerebellar peduncles. These include the inferior peduncle (restiform body), the middle peduncle (the brachium pontis) and the superior peduncle (brachium conjunctivum). The major afferent pathway connecting the cerebral cortex and the cerebellum is the cortico-pontine-cerebellar pathway. This pathway originates primarily from the motor cortex and projects to the ipsilateral pontine nuclei from where secondary fibres project mainly to the cortex of the neocerebellum. Other afferent pathways project to the cerebellum from structures in the brainstem such as the olive (olivo-cerebellar tract), the red nucleus (rubro-cerebellar tract), the reticular formation (reticulo-cerebellar tract), the mid-brain (tecto-cerebellar tract) and the cuneate nucleus (cuneo-cerebellar tract) as well as from the spinal cord (spino-cerebellar tracts).

Efferent pathways from the cerebellum originate almost entirely from the deep nuclei and project to many parts of the central nervous system, including the motor cortex (via the thalamus), the basal ganglia, red nucleus, brainstem, reticular formation and the vestibular nuclei. The feedback loop provided by the extensive afferent and efferent connections of the cerebellum give it the means to both monitor and modify motor activities taking place in various parts of the body to produce a smooth, coordinated motor action.

Diseases of the cerebellum

The major diseases of the cerebellum are listed in Table 5.4 (see pp. 122–3). The signs and symptoms of cerebellar dysfunction are generally the same, regardless of aetiology. In those disorders where the lesion is slowly progressive (for example, cerebellar tumour), however, symptoms of cerebellar disease tend to be much less severe than in conditions where the lesion develops acutely (for example, traumatic head injury, cerebrovascular accident and so on). In addition, considerable recovery from the effects of an acute lesion can usually be expected.

Clinical characteristics of ataxic dysarthria

As indicated above, ataxic dysarthria is associated with decomposition of complex movements arising from a breakdown in the coordinated action of the muscles of the speech production mechanism. In particular, inaccuracy of movement, irregular rhythm of repetitive movement, uncoordination, slowness of both individual and repetitive movements and hypotonia of affected muscles seem to be the principal neuromuscular deficits associated with cerebellar damage that underlie ataxic dysarthria.

The disrupted speech output exhibited by individuals with cerebellar lesions has often been termed 'scanning speech', a term probably first used by Charcot (1877). According to Charcot (1877), 'the words are as if measured or scanned: there is a pause after every syllable, and the syllables themselves are pronounced slowly' (p.192). The most predominant features of ataxic dysarthria include a breakdown in the articulatory and prosodic aspects of speech. According to Brown, Darley and Aronson (1970), the 10 deviant speech dimensions most characteristic of ataxic dysarthria can be divided into three clusters: articulatory inaccuracy, characterized by imprecision of consonant production, irregular articulatory breakdowns and distorted vowels; prosodic excess, characterized by excess and equal stress, prolonged phonemes, prolonged intervals and slow rate; and phonatory-prosodic insufficiency, characterized by harshness, monopitch and monoloudness. Brown et al. (1970) believed that the articulatory problems were the product of ataxia of the respiratory and oral-buccal-lingual musculature, and prosodic excess was thought by these authors to result from slow movements. The occurrence of phonatory-prosodic insufficiencies was attributed to the presence of hypotonia.

Table 5.4: Diseases of the cerebellum

Diseases	Example	General features
Chromosomal disorders	Trisomy	Diffuse hypotrophy of the cerebellum may be present which may be associated with either no clinical symptoms of cerebellar dysfunction through to marked limb ataxia.
Congenital anomalies	Cerebellar agenesis	Partial to almost total non-development of the cerebellum. May in some cases not be associated with any clinical evidence of cerebellar dysfunction. In other cases, however, a gait disturbance may be evident in addition to limb ataxia (especially involving the lower limbs) and dysarthria.
Demyelinating disorders	Multiple sclerosis	Usually associated with demyelination in a number of regions of the central nervous system including the cerebellum. Consequently, the dysarthria, if present, usually takes the form of a mixed dysarthria rather than purely an ataxic dysarthria. Paroxysmal ataxic dysarthria may occur as an early sign of multiple sclerosis.
Hereditary ataxias	Friedreich's ataxia	The most commonly encountered spinal form of hereditary ataxia. Pathological degeneration primarily involves the spinal cord with degeneration of neurones occurring in the spino-cerebellar tracts. Some degeneration of neurones in the dentate nucleus and brachium conjunctivum may also occur. The first clinical sign of the disease is usually clumsiness of gait. Later limb ataxia (especially involving the lower extremities) also occurs. A large percentage of cases also exhibit dysarthria and nystagmus and cognitive deficits.
Infections	Cerebellar abscess	Most frequently caused by purulent bacteria but can also occur with fungi. Cerebellar abscesses most frequently arise by direct extension from adjacent infected areas such as the mastoid process or from otologic disease.
Toxic metabolic and endocrine disorders	Exogenous toxins, for example, industrial solvents, heavy metals, carbon tetrachloride, etc.	Signs of cerebellar involvement usually associated with symptoms of diffuse involvements of the central nervous system following these intoxications rather than appearing in isolation to other neurological deficits.
	Enzyme deficiencies, for example, pyruvate dehydrogenase deficiency	Ataxia most marked in lower limbs.
	Hypothyroidism	Cretins show poor development of the cerebellum. Ataxia present in 20–30% of myxoedema cases.

Table 5.4: (contd)

Diseases	Example	General features
Trauma	Penetrating head wounds	May be associated with either mild slowly developing cerebellar dysfunction or rapid, severe cerebellar dysfunction.
Tumours	Medulloblastomas, astrocytomas and ependymomas	Primary tumours of the cerebellum occur more frequently in children than in adults. Medulloblastomas occur most commonly in the midline of the cerebellum in children and usually have a rapid course with a poor prognosis. Astrocytomas are more benign than medulloblastomas and generally occur in children of an older age group than medulloblastomas. Ependymomas are relatively slow growing and again are more common in children than adults.

Respiratory function in ataxic dysarthria

Perceptual correlates of respiratory inadequacy have been noted in a number of perceptual studies of ataxic dysarthria (Kluin et al., 1988; Chenery, Ingram and Murdoch, 1991). In a study of 16 subjects with ataxic dysarthria, Chenery et al. (1991) reported the presence of significantly reduced ratings of respiratory support for speech as well as a respiratory pattern characterized by sudden forced inspiratory and expiratory sighs. Kluin et al. (1988) documented subjective reports of audible inspiration in ataxic dysarthric speakers investigated in their laboratory.

Evidence is also available from physiological studies to suggest that speech breathing is disturbed in ataxic dysarthria. Murdoch, Chenery, Stokes and Hardcastle (1991) employed both spirometric and kinematic techniques to investigate the respiratory function of a group of 12 subjects with ataxic dysarthria associated with cerebellar disease. Their results showed that almost one half of the ataxic cases had vital capacities below the normal limits of variation. In addition, the ataxic dysarthric speakers also demonstrated unusual patterns of chest wall two-part contribution to lung volume change, including the presence of abdominal and ribcage paradoxing, abrupt changes in movements of the ribcage and abdomen and a tendency to initiate utterances at lower than normal lung volume levels. Murdoch et al. (1991) suggested that these findings were an outcome of impaired coordination of the chest wall and speculated that such respiratory anomalies had the potential to underlie some of the prosodic abnormalities observed in ataxic dysarthria.

Laryngeal function in ataxic dysarthria

Phonatory disturbances are frequently listed among the most deviant or most frequently occurring perceptually deviant speech dimensions in ataxic dysarthria (Brown et al., 1970; Darley et al., 1975; Enderby, 1986; Chenery et al., 1991). The perceptual features listed that can be attributed to laryngeal dysfunction in ataxic dysarthria include disorders of vocal quality (for example, a harsh voice, strained-strangled phonation, pitch breaks and vocal tremor), impairment of pitch level (for example, elevated or lower pitch), and deficits in variability of pitch and loudness (for example, monopitch, monoloudness and excess loudness variation). It should be noted that, as indicated by Darley et al. (1975), although attributed to phonatory dysfunction, many of the above speech deviations could also result, at least partly, from dysfunction at other levels of the speech production mechanism (for example, the respiratory system).

Unfortunately, only one study reported to date has used physiological instrumentation to investigate laryngeal activity in ataxic dysarthria. Grémy, Chevrie-Muller and Garde (1967) used electroglottography to identify increased variability of vocal fold vibrations in ataxic subjects.

Velopharyngeal function in ataxic dysarthria

The presence of hypernasal speech and nasal emission is not a commonly reported feature of ataxic dysarthria, suggesting that functioning of the velopharyngeal port may be normal in patients with cerebellar lesions. Duffy (1995) did report, however, that in some rare cases ataxic subjects may exhibit mild hyponasality, possibly as a consequence of improper timing of velar and articulatory gestures for nasal consonants. Oral examination of patients with cerebellar disorders most often reveals that elevation of the soft palate during phonation is normal.

Articulatory and prosodic function in ataxic dysarthria

The most prominent features of ataxic dysarthria involve a breakdown in articulatory and prosodic aspects of speech. The imprecise articulation leads to improper formation and separation of individual syllables leading to a reduction in intelligibility while the disturbance in prosody is associated with loss of texture, tone, stress and rhythm of individual syllables.

As indicated earlier, Brown et al. (1970) concluded that the 10 deviant speech dimensions perceived to be the most characteristic of ataxic dysarthria fell into three clusters: articulatory inaccuracy, prosodic excess, and phonatory-prosodic insufficiency. Based on the performance of ataxic speakers on the Frenchay Dysarthria Assessment (Enderby, 1983), Enderby (1986) also observed perceptual correlates of articulatory and prosodic inadequacy to be prominent among the 10 features she believed to be the most characteristic of ataxic dysarthria, including poor intonation, poor tongue movement in speech, poor alternating movement of the tongue in speech, reduced rate of speech, reduced lateral movement of the tongue, reduced elevation of the tongue, poor alternating movement of the lips and poor lip movements in speech.

In addition to the perceptual studies of ataxic dysarthria mentioned above, a number of researchers have used either acoustic and/or physiological procedures to study the articulatory and prosodic aspects of ataxic dysarthria. Kent, Netsell and Abbs (1979) examined the acoustic features of five patients with ataxic dysarthria. They reported that the most marked and consistent abnormalities observed in the spectrograms of these speakers were alterations in the normal timing patterns and a tendency towards equalized syllable durations. These authors concluded that general timing is a major problem in ataxic dysarthria. Further, they speculated that ataxic speakers fail to decrease syllable duration when appropriate because such reductions require flexibility in sequencing complex motor instructions. The lack of flexibility may lead to a syllable-by-syllable motor control strategy with subsequent abnormal stress patterns.

Only a few studies reported to date have used physiological instrumentation to investigate the functioning of the articulators in ataxic dysarthria. In support of the concept that ataxic speakers are impaired in motor control, McClean, Beukelman and Yorkston (1987) reported the case of an ataxic speaker who performed poorly on a non-speech visuo-motor tracking task involving the lower lip and jaw. Kent and Netsell (1975) and Netsell and Kent (1976) analysed articulatory position and movements in ataxic speakers using cineradiography. They observed a number of abnormal articulatory movements including abnormally small adjustments of anterior-posterior tongue movements during vowel production, which they thought may form the basis of the perception of vowel distortions. Although movements of the lips, tongue and jaw were generally coordinated, these authors reported that individual movements of these structures were often slow. In addition, they noted that articulatory contacts for consonant production were occasionally incomplete.

Hirose and colleagues (1978) used an X-ray microbeam technique and electromyography to investigate articulatory dynamics in two dysarthric patients, one of whom had cerebellar degeneration. In particular they examined the movement patterns in the jaw and lower lip. Their results showed that the ataxic speaker demonstrated inconsistency in articulatory movements, being characterized by inconsistency in both range and velocity of movement. Further, Hirose et al. (1978) found that electromyography evidenced a breakdown of rhythmic patterns in articulatory muscles during syllable repetition. Overall, the findings of Hirose et al. (1978) are consistent with the perception that ataxic speech contains irregular articulatory breakdowns.

In an examination of four ataxic speakers, McNeil and colleagues (1990) investigated isometric force and static position control of the upper and lower lip, tongue and jaw during non-speech tasks. They reported that the ataxic speakers had greater force and position instability than normal speakers, although impairment on one task did not necessarily predict impairment on other tasks.

Hypokinetic dysarthria

Neuroanatomical framework of hypokinetic dysarthria

As pointed out earlier in this chapter under the heading of 'spastic dysarthria', the descending motor pathways can be divided into two subsystems, one a direct system and the other an indirect system. The indirect system consists of a complex series of multi-synaptic pathways which indirectly connect the motor areas of the cerebral cortex to the level of the lower motor neurones and which has previously been called the 'extrapyramidal system'. The major components of the extrapyramidal system include the basal ganglia plus the various brain-stem nuclei that contribute to motor functioning. Diseases which selectively affect the extrapyramidal system without involving the pyramidal pathways are referred to as 'extrapyramidal syndromes' and include a number of clinically defined disease states of diverse aetiology and often obscure pathogenesis (for example, Parkinson's disease, chorea, athetosis and so on). Movement disorders are the primary features of extrapyramidal syndromes and, where the muscles of the speech mechanism are involved, disorders of speech may occur in the form of either hypokinetic or hyperkinetic dysarthria.

Neurological disorders associated with hypokinetic dysarthria

Darley et al. (1969a, b) first used the term 'hypokinetic dysarthria' to describe the speech disorder associated with Parkinson's disease. An acoustically similar form of dysarthria, however, has also been observed in persons with progressive supra-nuclear palsy (Steele-Richardson-Olszewski syndrome) (Metter and Hanson, 1986).

Parkinson's disease

Parkinson's disease (PD) is a progressive, degenerative, neurological disease associated with selective loss of dopaminergic neurones in the substantia nigra (Utti and Calne, 1993). A speech disorder may in some cases be the first symptom to emerge (Hoehn and Yahr, 1967). Gracco, Marek and Gracco (1993) and Hanson (1991) found laryngeal dysfunction to be readily observable in subjects with early PD, and indicated that it may precede the appearance of symptoms elsewhere. It has been estimated that 60–80% of patients with Parkinson's disease exhibit hypokinetic dysarthria, with the prevalence increasing as the disease advances (Scott, Caird and Williams, 1985; Johnson and Pring, 1990). Some authors have suggested that more than 75% of people with parkinsonism eventually develop speech and voice deficits that decrease their ability to communicate with family and friends and limit their employment opportunities (Oxtoby, 1982; Streifler and Hofman, 1984). Treatment of PD usually involves prescription of one of the L-dopa drugs such as Sinemet or Parlodel. Other treatment strategies being explored include surgical methods (for example, thalomotomy, pallidotomy) and restorative techniques (for example, brain implants, gene replacement therapy) (Stacy and Jankovic, 1993).

Progressive supra-nuclear palsy

Progressive supra-nuclear palsy is conventionally taken to refer to the subcortical degenerative syndrome first described by Steele, Richardson and Olszewski (1964). This is a progressive neurological disorder with onset usually occurring in middle to later life. Affected persons have an associated akinetic-rigid syndrome, pseudobulbar palsy and dementia of frontal type. At necropsy, neuronal loss with neurofibrillary tangle inclusions in a proportion of the remaining neurones, and gliosis are characteristically found in the basal ganglia, brainstem and cerebellar nuclei but not in the cerebral or cerebellar cortex. The initial symptoms of progressive supra-nuclear palsy have been described as feelings of unsteadiness, vague visual difficulties, speech problems and minor changes in personality. As the disease progresses, symptoms include supra-nuclear opthalmoplegia affecting chiefly vertical gaze, pseudobulbar palsy, dysarthria, dystonic rigidity of the neck and upper trunk and mild dementia as well as other cerebellar and pyramidal symptoms. The disease is rapidly progressive, resulting in marked incapacity of the patient in two to three years.

Patients with progressive supra-nuclear palsy tend to have mask-like faces and akinesia as seen in Parkinson's disease. They do not, however, exhibit tremor and have relatively good associated movements (for example, arm swinging when walking). Affected individuals have a peculiar erect posture with backward retraction of the neck. Although reported by Steele et al. (1964) to have only minimal rigidity in the extremities, these patients do have severe rigidity of the axial musculature, especially in the latter stages of the disorder. The aetiology of progressive supra-nuclear palsy is unknown.

Clinical characteristics of hypokinetic dysarthria

Features of the speech disorder seen in association with Parkinson's disease are frequently described as including a monotony of pitch and loudness, decreased use of all vocal parameters for effecting stress and emphasis, breathy and harsh vocal quality, reduced vocal intensity, variable rate including short rushes of speech or accelerated speech, consonant imprecision, impaired breath support for speech, reduction in phonation time, difficulty in the initiation of speech activities, and inappropriate silences (Darley et al., 1969a, b, 1975; Logemann et al., 1978; Critchley, 1981; Ludlow and Bassich, 1983, 1984; Scott et al., 1985; Chenery, Murdoch and Ingram, 1988).

The hypokinetic dysarthria resulting from Parkinson's disease has been the subject of extensive perceptual, acoustic, and physiological analyses in order to produce a definitive description of the speech disorder and provide a basis for treatment programming. Although various studies have identified impairment in all aspects of speech production (respiration, phonation, resonance, articulation and prosody) involving the various subsystems of the speech production mechanism, the individual with PD is most likely to exhibit disturbances of prosody, phonation and articulation (Darley et al., 1975; Logemann et al., 1978; Chenery et al., 1988; Zwirner and Barnes, 1992).

Respiratory function in hypokinetic dysarthria

A number of the perceptual features identified in hypokinetic dysarthria, such as a reduction in overall loudness, decay of loudness, reduced phrase length, short rushes of speech and reduced phonation time, have been attributed to the impairment of respiration (Canter, 1965; Darley et al., 1975). In support of these assumptions, Chenery et al. (1988) identified a mild impairment of respiratory support for speech in the majority (89%) of their subjects with PD. In addition, more than half of their subjects demonstrated reductions in phrase lengths, short rushes of speech, reduced loudness and decay of loudness during speech. Similarly, Ludlow and Bassich (1984) identified a reduction in overall loudness in 42% of their subjects, and the majority of their PD subjects demonstrated a variable rate of speech which could be partially attributed to respiratory insufficiency.

Significant reductions in the vital capacity of subjects with PD have been identified by several investigators (Cramer, 1940; De La Torre, Mier and Boshes, 1960; Laszewski, 1956). In particular, De La Torre et al. (1960) found that two-thirds of their subjects with PD recorded vital capacities 40% below the expected values, and Laszewski (1956) found that the majority of subjects exhibited a marked reduction in vital capacity, with little measurable thoracic excursion during inhalation or exhalation. During a sustained phonation task, Mueller (1971) found that PD subjects expended significantly smaller volumes of air than control subjects. Using spirographic analysis, Hovestadt and colleagues (1989) revealed that, on non-speech tasks, peak inspiratory and expiratory flow, and maximum expiratory flow at a 50% level were significantly below normal for subjects with relatively severe PD. In contrast, neither Murdoch et al. (1989) nor Solomon and Hixon (1993) identified significant overall reductions in vital capacity and lung volumes in their groups of subjects with PD.

Recent studies involving kinematic investigations of respiratory function in Parkinson's disease have also identified incoordination of the components of the chest wall during speech breathing. Murdoch et al. (1989) identified irregularities in chest wall movement during the production of sustained vowels and syllable repetitions. These abnormal chest wall movements took the form of abrupt changes in the relative contribution of the chest wall components and featured both ribcage and abdominal paradoxical movements. In addition, Murdoch et al. (1989) found that the PD subjects demonstrated a wide range of relative volume contributions of the ribcage and abdomen during speech breathing, with a predominance of ribcage involvement. Solomon and Hixon (1993), using different instrumentation, however, recorded smaller ribcage than abdominal contribution to lung volume change in the speech breathing of PD subjects and found that ribcage and abdominal paradoxing were not specific to PD subjects alone. Both studies, however, identified a significantly greater breathing rate and minute ventilation in the subjects with PD compared with the controls (Murdoch et al., 1993).

Laryngeal function in hypokinetic dysarthria

Phonatory disturbance is often the initial symptom of the ensuing speech disorder associated with PD. In fact, Logemann et al. (1978) identified laryngeal problems as being the most prominent deviant features in their group of 200 subjects with PD, occurring in 89% of cases. Similarly, about half of the deviant speech dimensions, identified by Darley et al. (1975) and Ludlow and Bassich (1983) as being the most distinguishing features of hypokinetic dysarthria, related to phonatory disturbance. The deviant perceptual features associated with laryngeal dysfunction in PD include disorders of vocal quality and impairment of the overall levels and variability of pitch and loudness.

Unfortunately, very few studies reported in the literature have been based on physiological investigation of laryngeal function in persons with Parkinson's disease. Collectively, those studies that have been reported have shown that individuals with PD demonstrate abnormal vocal fold posturing and vibratory patterns, and laryngeal aerodynamics (Hanson, Gerratt and Ward, 1983; Hirose, Sawashima and Niimi, 1985; Gerratt, Hanson and Berke, 1987; Murdoch et al., 1995).

Velopharyngeal function in hypokinetic dysarthria

Controversy surrounds the existence of a resonatory disturbance in persons with PD. Several authors have reported low incidences of perceived hypernasality in groups of PD subjects (Darley et al., 1975; Logemann et al., 1978; Hoodin and Gilbert, 1989a, b; Theodoros, Murdoch and Thompson, 1995). At the same time, hypernasality has been identified as one of the most useful perceptual features for differentiating between hypokinetic dysarthria and normal speech (Ludlow and Bassich, 1983). For some individuals, hypernasality has been found to be the most prominent deviant speech feature (Hoodin and Gilbert, 1989a, b).

Physiological evaluation of velopharyngeal function using a variety of direct and indirect instrumental techniques, has provided objective evidence of dysfunction of the velopharyngeal valve in subjects with PD. Hirose and colleagues (1981) conducted a study in which velar movements were directly observed by means of an X-ray microbeam system that tracked a lead pellet attached to the nasal side of the velum. During the rapid repetition of the monosyllable /ten/, Hirose et al. (1981) identified a gradual decrease in the degree of displacement of the velum. In effect, the lowering and elevation of the velum for the nasal and non-nasal consonants, respectively, were found to be incomplete towards the end of the speech task. At a rapid rate of repetition, the interval between each utterance was noted to be inconsistent and the displacement and rate of velar movements were found to be markedly reduced (Hirose et al., 1981).

In a study involving the use of videofluoroscopy to examine velar movements during speech in subjects with PD, Robbins, Logemann and Kirshner (1986) identified a significant reduction in velar elevation, which was considered to reflect a reduced range of velar movement. Nasal accelerometry has also revealed a significantly greater degree and frequency of increased nasality in the speech output of a group of hypokinetic speakers with PD (Theodoros et al., 1995). Specifically, the PD subjects, as a group, recorded significantly higher Horii Oral Nasal Coupling (HONC) Indices compared with the controls. Of the 23 PD subjects, 17 (74%) were identified as exhibiting increased nasality.

Articulatory function in hypokinetic dysarthria

By far the majority of speakers with hypokinetic dysarthria exhibit disorders of articulation. Articulatory impairments such as consonant and vowel imprecision and prolongation of phonemes have been observed, with consonant imprecision identified as the most common articulatory disturbance (Darley et al., 1975, Logemann et al., 1978; Chenery et al., 1988; Zwirner and Barnes, 1992). Consonant articulation has been found to be characterized by errors in the manner of production involving incomplete closure for stops and partial constriction of the vocal tract for fricatives, resulting in the abnormal production of stop-plosives, affricates and fricatives (Canter, 1965; Logemann and Fisher, 1981).

In addition to abnormalities of articulation, disordered speech rate is also frequently observed in patients with PD. Perceptually, individuals with PD have been noted to demonstrate both a faster (Darley et al., 1975; Critchley, 1981; Enderby, 1986; Chenery et al., 1988; Zwirner and Barnes, 1992) and a slower overall rate of speech than normal (Chenery et al., 1988; Zwirner and Barnes, 1992), with most studies suggesting that the speech rate of these patients is generally variable (Ludlow and Bassich, 1983, 1984; Scott et al., 1985; Netsell, 1986; Hoodin and Gilbert, 1989a). In addition, subjects with PD have been noted to demonstrate short rushes of speech, or what is perceived as an 'accelerated' speech pattern (Darley et al., 1975; Netsell, Daniel and Celesia, 1975; Scott et al., 1985; Chenery et al., 1988; Zwirner and Barnes, 1992). The production of short rushes of speech in the verbal output of speakers with PD was found by Darley et al. (1975) to be one of the most prominent features of hypokinetic dysarthria. Furthermore, this deviant speech dimension was identified in 84% of the subjects assessed in the study by Chenery et al. (1988). In some cases, a progressive acceleration of speech within a speech segment has also been perceived to be present (Selby, 1968; Scott et al., 1985; Chenery et al., 1988).

Physiological investigations of the articulatory function of patients with Parkinson's disease have identified the presence of abnormal patterns of muscle activity, reductions in the range and velocity of articulatory movement, impaired strength, endurance and fine force control of the articulators and tremor in the orofacial structures. These investigations have included a wide variety of instrumental techniques including direct recordings of muscle activity such as electromyography (Hunker, Abbs and Barlow, 1982; Hirose, 1986; Moore and Scudder, 1989) and a range of kinematic procedures, including strain-gauge transduction systems (Abbs, Hunker and Barlow, 1983; Connor et al., 1989), lead-pellet tracking (Hirose, Kiritani and Sawashima, 1982a; Hirose, 1986), electromagnetic articulography (Ackermann et al., 1993) and optoelectrics (Svensson, Henningson and Karlsson, 1993).

Prosodic function in hypokinetic dysarthria

According to Darley et al. (1975), prosodic disturbances constitute the most prominent features of hypokinetic dysarthria. Descriptions of the speech of persons with PD frequently refer to the dysprosodic aspects of speech production in relation to stress and intonation, fluency and rate. Impairment of stress patterning, variable rate, short rushes of speech or 'accelerated' speech, difficulty in the initiation of speech, phoneme repetition, palilalia, inappropriate silences, and monotony of pitch and loudness have been identified in these individuals (Darley et al., 1975; Critchley, 1981; Ludlow and Bassich, 1983, 1984; Scott and Caird, 1983; Netsell, 1986; Chenery et al., 1988; Zwirner and Barnes, 1992).

Hyperkinetic dysarthria

Neuroanatomical framework of hyperkinetic dysarthria

Hyperkinetic dysarthria occurs in association with a variety of extrapyramidal syndromes in which the deviant speech characteristics are the product of abnormal involuntary movements which disturb the rhythm and rate of motor activities. Although known to be associated with dysfunction of the basal ganglia, the underlying neural mechanisms by which these abnormal involuntary movements are produced are poorly understood. Anatomically, the basal ganglia consist of the caudate nucleus, the putamen, the globus pallidus and the amygdaloid nucleus. Some neurologists also include another nucleus, the claustrum, as part of the basal ganglia. Although a number of brainstem nuclei, including the subthalamic nuclei, the substantia nigra and the red nucleus are functionally related to the basal ganglia, they are not anatomically part of it. Collectively, the globus pallidus and the putamen are referred to as the lenticular nucleus (lentiform nucleus).

Neurological disorders associated with hyperkinetic dysarthria

Any process that damages the basal ganglia or related brain structures has the potential to cause hyperkinetic dysarthria including degenerative, vascular, traumatic, inflammatory, toxic and metabolic disorders. In some cases the cause of hyperkinetic dysarthria is idiopathic. The major types of hyperkinetic disorders are outlined in Table 5.5 (see pp. 134–5).

Mixed dysarthria

A number of disorders of the nervous system affect more than one level of the motor system. Consequently, although pure forms of dysarthria do occur, mixed dysarthria, involving a combination of two or more types of dysarthria, is often exhibited by neurological cases referred to speech pathology clinics. A variety of neurological disorders can cause mixed dysarthria, including central nervous system degenerative diseases (for example, amyotrophic lateral sclerosis, Wilson's disease), cerebrovascular accidents, traumatic brain injury, demyelinating disorders, brain tumours, and toxic-metabolic and inflammatory diseases. As examples, three neurological diseases that typically display symptoms of mixed dysarthria are described here, including amyotrophic lateral sclerosis, multiple sclerosis and Wilson's disease.

Amyotrophic lateral sclerosis

Amyotrophic lateral sclerosis (ALS) is a form of motor neurone disease characterized by a selective and progressive degeneration in the cortico-spinal and cortico-bulbar pathways and in the motor neurones associated with the cranial nerves and anterior horn cells of the spinal cord. The aetiology of ALS has to date not been determined, although there is evidence to suggest that immunological and metabolic disturbances may contribute to the manifestation of the disease (Sadiq et al., 1990; Specola et al., 1990).

The clinical features of ALS include muscle weakness and atrophy which are often asymmetric and sporadic, fasciculations, cramps, dysarthria, dysphagia, fatigue, spasticity, emotional lability, hyper-reflexia, and progressive respiratory impairment (Rowland, 1980; Tandan, 1994) while less typical features include oculomotor dysfunction, sensory abnormalities, and autonomic nervous system involvement (Tandan, 1994).

Table 5.5: Major types of hyperkinetic disorder

Disorder	Symptoms	Effect on speech
Myoclonic jerks	Characterized by abrupt, sudden, unsustained muscle contractions which occur irregularly. Involuntary contractions may occur as single jerks of the body or may be repetitive. Two forms may affect speech – palatal myoclonus and action myoclonus.	Speech disorder in palatal myoclonus usually characterized by phonatory, resonatory and prosodic abnormalities, for example, vocal tremor, rhythmic phonatory arrests, intermittent hypernasality, prolonged intervals and inappropriate silences.
Tics	Gilles de la Tourette's syndrome characterized by development of motor and vocal tics plus behavioural disorders. Vocal tics include simple vocal tics (for example, , grunting, coughing, barking, hissing, etc.) and complex vocal tics (for example, stuttering-like repetitions, palilalia, echolalia and coprolalia). Brief, unsustained, recurrent, compulsive movements. Usually involve a small part of the body, for example, facial grimace.	Action myoclonus – speech disrupted as a result of fine, arrhythmic, erratic muscle jerks, triggered by activity of the speech musculature.
Chorea	A choreic movement consists of a single, involuntary, unsustained, isolated muscle action producing a short, rapid, uncoordinated jerk of the trunk, limb, face, tongue, diaphragm, etc. Contractions are random in distribution and timing is irregular. Two major forms – Sydenham's and Huntington's chorea.	A perceptual study of 30 patients with chorea demonstrated deficits in all aspects of speech production (Darley et al., 1969a). Physiological studies of the speech disturbance in chorea are as yet unreported.
Ballism	Rare hyperkinetic disorder characterized by involuntary, wide-amplitude, vigorous, flailing movements of the limbs. Facial muscles may also be affected.	Least important hyperkinetic disorders with regard to occurrence of hyperkinetic dysarthria.

Table 5.5: (contd)

Disorder	Symptoms	Effect on speech
Athetosis	Slow hyperkinetic disorder characterized by continuous, arrhythmic, purposeless, slow, writhing-type movements that tend to flow one into another. Muscles of the face, neck and tongue are involved, leading to facial grimacing, protrusion and writhing of the tongue and problems with speaking and swallowing.	Descriptions of the speech disturbance in athetosis largely related to athetoid cerebral palsy rather than hyperkinetic dysarthria in adults.
Dyskinesia	Two dyskinetic disorders are included under this heading: tardive dyskinesia and Levodopa-induced dyskinesia. Basic pattern of abnormal involuntary movement in both of these conditions is one of slow, repetitive, writhing, twisting, flexing and extending movements often with a mixture of tremor. Muscles of the tongue, face and oral cavity most often affected.	Accurate placement of the articulators of speech may be severely hampered by the presence of choreoathetoid movements of the tongue, lip pursing and smacking, tongue protrusion and sucking and chewing behaviours.
Dystonia	Characterized by abnormal involuntary movements that are slow and sustained for prolonged periods of time. Involuntary movements tend to have an undulant, sinuous character that may produce grotesque posturing and bizarre writhing, twisting movements.	Dystonias affecting the speech mechanism may result in respiratory irregularities and/or abnormal movement and bizarre posturing of the jaw, lips, tongue, face and neck. In particular, focal cranial/orolingual-mandibular dystonia and spasmodic torticollis have the most direct effect on speech function.

The presence of a severe speech disorder is a common finding in ALS, usually in the form of a mixed flaccid-spastic dysarthria. However, the speech disturbance may not always present as mixed throughout the course of the disease. It is possible that initially the dysarthria will present as either flaccid or spastic with a predominance of either type as the disease progresses (Duffy, 1995). For those patients where upper motor neurone involvement predominates, the dysarthric speech disturbance is associated with spasticity of the tongue, the presence of primitive reflexes, and emotional lability, consistent with pseudobulbar palsy (Gallagher, 1989). Bulbar dysfunction resulting in dysarthria and/or dysphagia has been found to occur in most individuals with ALS (Bonduelle, 1975; Dworkin and Hartman, 1979). The clinical signs of the dysarthria resulting from predominantly lower motor neurone involvement (bulbar palsy) consist of fasciculations, weakness, atrophy, and reduced mobility of the tongue, and lip and jaw muscle dysfunction (DePaul et al., 1988; Tandan, 1994). Swallowing and chewing difficulties are closely associated with the presentation of dysarthria (Robbins, 1987), particularly in those patients with bulbar palsy, and reflect the neurological involvement of the tongue (force and coordination), pharynx and jaw musculature (Tandan, 1994).

Multiple sclerosis

Multiple sclerosis (MS) is the most common primary demyelinating disease and is a major cause of neurological disability in young adults in most western countries. The disease tends to vary in incidence and prevalence across different regions of the world, being most common in the temperate areas of the world and rare in the tropics. In about two-thirds of cases the condition is characterized by periods of exacerbation and remission so that the course of the disease is variable. In the remaining one-third, the course of the disorder is progressive without remissions.

Neuropathologically, MS manifests in the form of irregular grey islands known as 'plaques' scattered throughout the white matter of the central nervous system, including the cerebrum, brainstem, cerebellum and spinal cord (Van Oosten et al., 1995). The plaques represent areas of demyelination of nerve fibres, although the axons and neurone cell bodies remain relatively well preserved (Murdoch, 1990). As yet the aetiology of MS is undetermined, although a number of possible explanations have been proposed.

Due to the disseminated neuropathology that may occur in MS, the clinical signs and symptoms of the disease are highly variable. A multitude of abnormal motor, sensory, cranial nerve/brainstem, cognitive and autonomic nervous system features exhibited by individuals have been described. Dysarthria is the most common communication disorder affecting individuals with MS (Beukelman, Kraft and Freal,

1985), occurring in about 47% of the MS population. Despite Charcot's (1877) inclusion of dysarthria in the triad of symptoms considered to be pathognomic of the disease, this speech disturbance is now not regarded as a consistent feature of MS. Darley, Brown and Goldstein (1972), in a study of 168 patients with MS, found that only 41% of these individuals exhibited some form of deviant speech behaviour, with the majority of patients (28%) demonstrating a mild speech impairment. A similar incidence of dysarthria was noted by Hartelius, Svensson and Bubach (1993) in a group of 30 subjects, 47% of whom were dysarthric. Surveys of MS populations, conducted by Beukelman et al. (1985) and Hartelius and Svensson (1994), have reported incidences of speech disturbances in 23% and 44% of respondents, respectively. The severity of dysarthria in individuals with MS would seem to be mild initially, with an increase in speech impairment corresponding to an increase in the overall severity of the disease, the number of neurological systems involved and the general deterioration in functioning of the individual (Darley et al., 1972; Beukelman et al., 1985). Indeed, the dysarthria associated with MS can be severe enough to warrant augmentative communication (Beukelman et al., 1985).

Given the potential of central nervous system involvement in MS, it is generally accepted that the dysarthria associated with MS is predominantly mixed, although specific types of dysarthria may present in some individuals at various stages of the disease. The type of dysarthria exhibited by the individual will be dependent, therefore, on the sites of demyelination. Duffy (1995) concluded that, based on perceptual evidence and knowledge of neurological involvement (Darley et al., 1972; Farmakides and Boone, 1960), ataxic and spastic dysarthria and a mixed ataxic-spastic dysarthria were the most frequently observed forms of dysarthria demonstrated by individuals with MS, although any other types or combinations of dysarthria may present in association with the disease.

Wilson's disease

Wilson's disease, or hepato-lenticular degeneration, is a rare, inborn metabolic disorder involving an inability to process dietary copper. As a result, copper builds up in the tissues of the liver, brain (especially the basal ganglia) and cornea of the eyes. The first symptoms of the disease typically occur in late adolescence or early adulthood, at about 15 to 17 years of age (Stremmel et al., 1991).

The clinical presentation of Wilson's disease includes neurological, hepatic, haematological, and, in some cases, psychiatric symptoms (Denning and Berrios, 1989; Adams and Victor, 1991; Oder et al., 1991; Stremmel et al., 1991). The most common clinical signs and symptoms of the disease identified by investigators have included mainly parkinsonian and hyperkinetic neurological behaviours. Stremmel et al.

(1991), in a group of 51 subjects with Wilson's disease, included dysarthria, tremor, writing difficulties, ataxic gait, hepatomegaly, splenomegaly and thombocytopenia, while other investigators have reported the presence of dysdiadochokinesis, dystonia, rigidity, facial masking, wing-beating tremor, bradykinesia, dysphagia, drooling, and gait and postural abnormalities (Adams and Victor, 1991; Oder et al., 1991).

Dysarthria is considered to be a characteristic feature of Wilson's disease and has been reported to occur in 51–81% of patients (Martin, 1968; Starosta-Rubinstein et al., 1987; Oder et al., 1991; Stremmel et al., 1991). The disordered speech takes the form of a mixed dysarthria consisting of mainly spastic, ataxic and hypokinetic components (Duffy, 1995). Starosta-Rubinstein et al. (1987) identified a predominance of spastic dysarthric components in the mixed dysarthria exhibited by their subjects, occurring in 76%, while features of ataxic dysarthria and hypokinetic dyarthria were evident in 69% and 59%, respectively. Slow hyperkinetic dystonia has also been observed in these patients to varying degrees (Starosta-Rubinstein et al., 1987). The combination of dysarthria types and the level of severity varies widely among individuals with the disease (Berry et al., 1974).

To date, there have been very few investigations of the dysarthric speech disturbance evident in patients with Wilson's disease. While the perceptual characteristics of the disturbed speech have been addressed to some extent (Berry et al., 1974), no studies have endeavoured to define the physiological and acoustic features of the dysarthric speech disturbance in this population.

Assessment of dysarthria

Techniques available for assessing dysarthric speech for the purposes of differential diagnosis and determination of treatment priorities can be broadly divided into three major categories. These include: perceptual techniques – these assessments are based on the clinician's impression of the auditory-perceptual attributes of the speech; acoustic techniques – assessments in this category are based on the study of the generation, transmission and modification of sound waves emitted from the vocal tract; physiological techniques – these methods are based on instrumental assessment of the functioning of the various subsystems of the speech production apparatus in terms of their movements, muscular contractions, biomechanical activities and so on.

Perceptual assessment

In the past years, perceptual analysis of dysarthric speech has been the 'gold standard' and preferred method by which clinicians made differential diagnoses and defined treatment programmes for their dysarthric clients. In fact, many clinicians have relied almost exclusively on auditory-perceptual judgements of speech intelligibility, articulatory accuracy or subjective ratings of various speech dimensions on which to base their diagnosis of dysarthric speech and plan their intervention. The use of auditory-perceptual assessment to characterize the different types of dysarthria and to identify the spectrum of deviant speech characteristics associated with each was pioneered by Darley et al. (1969a, b, 1975). As indicated earlier, it was from the findings of their auditory-perceptual studies of dysarthria that the system of classification of dysarthria most frequently used in clinical settings and used throughout the present chapter, was developed. Darley et al. (1969a, b) assessed speech samples taken from 212 dysarthric speakers with a variety of neurological conditions on 38 speech dimensions which fell into seven categories: pitch, loudness, voice quality (including both laryngeal and resonatory dysfunction), respiration, prosody, articulation and two summary dimensions relating to intelligibility and bizarreness. A key component of their research was the application of the 'equal-appearing intervals scale of severity', which used a seven-part scale of severity. In addition to rating scales, other perceptual assessments used to investigate dysarthric speech include application of intelligibility measures, phonetic transcription studies and articulation inventories. A full description of these methods is beyond the scope of the present chapter; however, the reader is referred to an excellent review of perceptual techniques by Chenery (1998).

The major advantages of perceptual assessment are those that have led to its preferred use as the tool for characterizing and diagnosing dysarthric speech. Perceptual assessments are readily available and require only limited financial outlay. In addition, all students of speech/language pathology are taught how to test for and identify perceptual symptoms. Enderby (1983) reported good discrimination ability (90% accuracy) of the perceptual dimensions rated in the Frenchay Dysarthria Assessment when differentiating subgroups of dysarthria. Finally, perceptual assessments are useful for monitoring the effects of treatment on speech intelligibility and the adequacy of communication.

Clinicians need to be aware, however, that there are a number of inherent inadequacies with perceptual assessment that may limit their use in determining treatment priorities. First, accurate, reliable perceptual judgements are often difficult to achieve as they can be influenced by a number of factors including the skill and experience of the clinician and the sensitivity of the assessment (Chenery, 1998). As pointed out by Rosenbek and LaPointe (1978), raters must have extensive structured experience in listening prior to performing perceptual ratings.

Second, perceptual assessments are difficult to standardize both in relation to the patient being rated and the environment in which the speech samples are recorded. Patient variability over time and across different settings prevents maintenance of adequate intra- and inter-rater reliability (Ludlow and Bassich, 1983). Further, the symptoms may be present in certain conditions and not in others. This variability is also found in the patients themselves such that characteristics of the person being rated (for example, their age, premorbid medical history and social history) may influence speech as well as the neurological problem itself (Rosenbek and LaPointe, 1978).

A third factor that limits reliance on perceptual assessments is that certain speech symptoms may influence the perception of others (Rosenbek and LaPointe, 1978). This confound has been well reported in relation to the perception of resonatory disorders (for example, Brancewicz and Reich, 1989; Hoodin and Gilbert, 1989b), articulatory deficits (for example, Rosenbek and LaPointe, 1978; Ludlow and Bassich, 1983) and prosodic disturbances (for example, Lethlean, Chenery and Murdoch, 1990).

Probably the major concern of perceptual assessments, particularly as they relate to treatment planning, is that they have restricted power for determining which subsystems of the speech motor system are affected (Rosenbek and LaPointe, 1978; Ludlow and Bassich, 1983). In other words, perceptual assessments are unable to accurately identify the pathophysiological basis of the speech disorder manifest in various types of dysarthria. It is possible that a number of different physiological deficits can form the basis of perceptually identified features, and that different patterns of interaction within a patient's overall symptom complex can result in a similar perceptual deviation (for example, distorted consonants can result from reduced respiratory support for speech, from inadequate velopharyngeal functioning or from weak tongue musculature). When crucial decisions are required in relation to optimum therapeutic planning, an over-reliance on only perceptual assessment may lead to a number of questionable therapy directions.

Acoustic assessment

Acoustic analyses can be used in conjunction with perceptual assessments to provide a more complete understanding of the nature of the disturbance in dysarthric speech. In particular, acoustic assessment can highlight aspects of the speech signal that may be contributing to the perception of deviant speech production and can provide confirmatory support for perceptual judgements. For example, they may confirm the perception that speech rate is slow and demonstrate that the reduced rate of speech may be the result of increased inter-word durations and prolonged vowel and consonant production. As a further example, an acoustic analysis might be used to confirm the perception of imprecise consonant production and to show that such imprecision is the result of spirantization of consonants and reduction of consonant clusters. In addition to altered speech rate and consonant imprecision, other perceived deviant speech dimensions that can be confirmed by way of acoustic analysis include, among others, breathy voice, voice tremor, and reduced variability of pitch and loudness. Acoustic analysis is also useful for providing objective documentation of the effects of treatment and disease progression on speech production (King et al., 1994; Ramig et al., 1994).

Acoustic measurements can be taken primarily from two different types of acoustic displays: oscillographic displays and spectrographic displays (Weismer, 1984). An oscillographic display is a two-dimensional waveform display of amplitude (on the y-axis) as a function of time (x-axis). Oscillographic displays are easy to generate and can provide information on a variety of acoustic parameters such as segment duration (for example, vowel duration, word duration and so on), amplitude, fundamental frequency, and the presence of some acoustic cues of articulatory adequacy such as voice onset time, spirantization, and voiced versus voiceless distinctions. Measurements from oscillographic displays can be made either manually or alternatively, by using computer-controlled acoustic analysis software.

In contrast to the two-dimensional oscillographic display, a spectrographic display is actually a three-dimensional display, of both frequency and amplitude as a function of time, where time is on the x-axis and frequency is displayed on the y-axis (Weismer, 1984). There are two different types of spectrographic displays: wide-band displays (also called broad-band displays) and narrow-band displays. Wide-band spectrographic displays are used to determine accurate temporal measurements, and narrow-band spectrograms are useful for making measurements of fundamental frequency and the prosodic aspects of speech.

While there is no 'standard' set of parameters included in all acoustic analyses, there are, however, a number of different acoustic measures which can provide important information about the acoustic features of dysarthric speech. These parameters can be loosely arranged into groups of measures, including fundamental frequency measures, amplitude measures, perturbation measures, noise-related measures, formant measures, temporal measures, measures of articulatory capability, and evaluations of manner of voicing.

Physiological assessment

Traditional therapeutic approaches to the rehabilitation of dysarthric speech are based primarily on subjective, perceptual assessments and techniques. Some clinicians believe that such methods lack the objectivity and specificity required to ensure the most effective rehabilitation, especially given the acknowledged inability of perceptual assessment to provide information regarding the pathophysiological basis of the speech disorder. What is needed is a more objective, physiological approach to dysarthria therapy – one that is based on a comprehensive instrumental assessment of the functioning of the subsystems of the speech production apparatus. Such an approach, often referred to as the physiological approach, has been advocated by Hardy (1967) and Netsell and colleagues (Netsell and Daniel, 1979; Netsell, 1986; Netsell, Lotz and Barlow, 1989).

The physiological approach to dysarthria rehabilitation is based on the concept that assessment of the individual motor subsystems of the speech mechanism (that is, respiratory, laryngeal, velopharyngeal and articulatory subsystems) is crucial in defining the underlying speech motor pathophysiology necessary for the development of optimal treatment programmes (Abbs and DePaul, 1989; Netsell, 1986). Therefore, in this approach the initial step is to undertake a comprehensive physiological assessment of the various components of the speech production mechanism of the dysarthric speaker to determine: first, those components that are malfunctioning and, second, the physiological nature and severity of the malfunction. Essentially, the goal of the physiological assessment is to evaluate the integrity of the speech components (for example, lips, tongue, jaw, velopharynx, larynx and so on) and systems (for example, articulation, phonation, respiration and so on) that generate or valve the expiratory airstream, and subsequently relate this information to the perceived dysarthric symptom (Kearns and Simmons, 1990). Whereas perceptual and acoustic assessments focus on the signal emitted from the vocal tract, physiological assessments analyse muscle contractions and movements within the speech mechanism and address whether specific deviant speech dimensions are the outcome of factors such as muscle weakness, spasticity and so on.

A wide variety of different types of instrumentation have been described in the literature for use in the assessment of the functioning of the various components of the speech production apparatus. Each of these instruments has been designed to provide information on a specific aspect of speech production, including muscular activity, structural movements, airflows and air pressures generated in the various parts of the speech mechanism. It is, however, beyond the scope of the present chapter to review all of the types of instrumentation available or go into the specific details of the instrumental techniques. For a comprehensive review of instrumental assessment of the speech mechanism the reader is referred to Thompson-Ward and Murdoch (1998).

In summary, although instrumentation has opened a whole new range of assessment techniques, physiological data should be integrated with data from other appraisal procedures (that is, combined information from perceptual, physiological, and acoustic procedures) to ensure that an accurate diagnosis is made and that the subsequent remediation techniques are appropriate. In particular, the limitations of each of the instrumental procedures need to be kept in mind when making clinical decisions based on their findings. It also must be remembered that despite the wide variety of objective instrumental measures available for documenting the physiology of speech production, to date, the clinical application of these techniques has been limited. Increasing the use of instrumentation in the clinical setting, for the purposes of both assessment and treatment, will require the implementation of training programmes for the clinicians as well as an increase in clinical research projects designed to demonstrate the clinical utility of instrumental techniques and to validate the role of instrumentation in dysarthria management.

References

Abbs JH, DePaul R (1989). Assessment of dysarthria: the critical prerequisite to treatment. In Leahy MM (ed.) Disorders of Communication: The Science of Intervention. London: Taylor and Francis, pp.206–27.

Abbs JH, Hunker CJ, Barlow SH (1983). Differential speech motor subsystem impairment with suprabulbar lesions: neurophysiological framework and supporting data. In Berry WR (ed.) Clinical Dysarthria. San Diego, CA: College Hill Press, pp.21–56.

Ackermann H, Grone BF, Hoch G, Schonle PW (1993). Speech freezing in Parkinson's disease: a kinematic analysis of orofacial movements by means of electromagnetic articulography. Folia Phoniatrica 45: 84–9.

Adams RD, Victor M (1991). Principles of Neurology. New York: McGraw-Hill.

Aten JA (1983). Treatment of Spastic Dysarthria. In Perkins W (ed.) Dysarthria and Apraxia. New York: Thieme-Stratton, pp.69–77.

Berry WR, Darley FL, Aronson AE, Goldstein NP (1974). Dysarthria in Wilson's disease. Journal of Speech and Hearing Research 17: 169–83.

Beukelman DR, Kraft GH, Freal J (1985). Expressive communication disorders in persons with multiple sclerosis: a survey. Archives of Physical Medicine and Rehabilitation 66: 675–7.

Bonduelle M (1975). Amyotrophic lateral sclerosis. In Vinken PJ and Bruyn GW (eds) Handbook of Clinical Neurology. Amsterdam: Elsevier, pp. 281–338.

Brancewicz TM, Reich AR (1989). Speech rate reduction and nasality in normal speakers. Journal of Speech and Hearing Research 32: 837–48.

Brown JR, Darley FL, Aronson AE (1970). Ataxic dysarthria. International Journal of Neurology 7: 302–18.

Canter G (1965). Speech characteristics of patients with Parkinson's disease. II. Physiological support for speech. Journal of Speech and Hearing Disorders 30: 44–9.

Charcot JM (1877). Lectures on the Diseases of the Nervous System. London: New Sydenham Society.

Chenery HJ (1998). Perceptual analysis of dysarthric speech. In Murdoch BE (ed.) Dysarthria: A Physiological Approach to Assessment and Ttreatment. Cheltenham: Stanley Thornes, pp.36–67.

Chenery HJ, Ingram JCL, Murdoch BE (1991). Perceptual analysis of speech in ataxic dysarthria. Australian Journal of Human Communication Disorders 18: 19–28.

Chenery HJ, Murdoch BE, Ingram JCL (1988). Studies in Parkinson's disease. I. Perceptual speech analysis. Australian Journal of Human Communication Disorders 16: 17–29.

Chenery HJ, Murdoch BE, Ingram JCL (1992). The perceptual speech characteristics of persons with pseudobulbar palsy. Australian Journal of Human Communication Disorders 20: 21–31.

Connor NP, Abbs JJ, Cole KJ, Gracco VL (1989). Parkinsonian deficits in serial multiarticulate movements for speech. Brain 112: 997–1009.

Cramer W (1940). De spraak bij patienten met Parkinsonisme. Logepaedie en Phoniatrie 22: 17–23.

Critchley EMR (1981). Speech disorders of Parkinsonism: a review. Journal of Neurology, Neurosurgery, and Psychiatry 44: 751–8.

Darley FL, Aronson AE, Brown JR (1969a). Differential diagnostic patterns of dysarthria. Journal of Speech and Hearing Research 12: 246–69.

Darley FL, Aronson AE, Brown JR (1969b). Clusters of deviant speech dimensions in the dysarthrias. Journal of Speech and Hearing Research 12: 462–96.

Darley FL, Aronson AE, Brown JR (1975). Motor Speech Disorders. Philadelphia, PA: WB Saunders.

Darley FL, Brown JR, Goldstein NP (1972). Dysarthria in multiple sclerosis. Journal of Speech and Hearing Research 15: 229–45.

De La Torre R, Mier M, Boshes B (1960). Studies in Parkinsonism: IX. Evaluation of respiratory function – preliminary observations. Quarterly Bulletin of The Northwestern University Medical School 34: 232–6.

Denning TR, Berrios GE (1989). Wilson's disease: a prospective study of psychopathology in 31 cases. British Journal of Psychiatry 155: 206–13.

DePaul R, Abbs JH, Caligiuri M, Gracco VL, Brooks BR (1988). Hypoglossal, trigeminal, and facial motoneuron involvement in amyotrophic lateral sclerosis. Neurology 38: 281–3.

Duffy JR (1995). Motor Speech Disorders: Substrates, Diagnosis and Management. St Louis, MO: Mosby.

Dworkin JP, Hartman DE (1979). Progressive speech deterioration and dysphagia in amyotrophic lateral sclerosis: case report. Archives of Physical Medicine and Rehabilitation 60: 423–5.

Enderby P (1983). Frenchay Dysarthria Assessment. San Diego, CA: College Hill Press.

Enderby P (1986). Relationships between dysarthric groups. British Journal of Disorders of Communication 21: 180–97.

Farmakides MN, Boone DR (1960). Speech problems of patients with multiple sclerosis. Journal of Speech and Hearing Disorders 25: 385–90.

Gallagher JP (1989). Pathologic laughter and crying in ALS: a search for their origin. Acta Neurologica Scandinavia 80: 114–17.

Gerratt,BR, Hanson DG, Berke GS (1987). Glottographic measures of laryngeal function in individuals with abnormal motor control. In Baer T, Sasaki C, Harris K (eds) Laryngeal Function in Phonation and Respiration. Boston, MA: College Hill Press, pp.521–31.

Gracco LC, Marek KL, Gracco VL (1993). Laryngeal manifestations of early Parkinson's disease: imaging and acoustic data. Neurology 43(Supplement 2): A285.

Grémy F, Chevrie-Muller C, Garde E (1967). Etude phoniatrique clinique et instrumentale des dysarthries. Review Neurologique 116: 401–26.

Hanson DG (1991). Neuromuscular disorders of the larynx. Otolaryngolgic Clinics of North America 24: 1035–51.

Hanson DG, Gerratt BR, Ward PH (1983). Glottographic measurement of vocal dysfunction: a preliminary report. Annals Otology, Rhinology, and Laryngology 92: 413–20.

Hardy JC (1967). Suggestions for physiological research in dysarthria. Cortex 3: 128–56.

Hartelius L, Svensson P (1994). Speech and swallowing symptoms associated with Parkinson's disease and multiple sclerosis: a survey. Folia Phonaiatrica 46: 9–17.

Hartelius L, Svensson P, Bubach A (1993). Clinical assessment of dysarthria: performance on a dysarthria test by normal adult subjects, and by individuals with Parkinson's disease or with multiple sclerosis. Scandinavian Journal of Logopedics and Phoniatrics 18: 131–41.

Hirose H (1986). Pathophysiology of motor speech disorders (dysarthria). Folia Phoniatrica 38: 61–88.

Hirose H, Kiritani S, Sawashima M (1980). Patterns of dysarthric movements in patients with amyotrophic lateral sclerosis and pseudobulbar palsy. Annual Bulletin of the Research Institute of Logopaedics and Phoniatrics 14: 263–72.

Hirose J, Kiritani S, Sawashima M (1982a). Patterns of dysarthric movement in patients with amyotrophic lateral sclerosis and pseudobulbar palsy. Folia Phoniatrica 34: 106–12.

Hirose H, Kiritani S, Sawashima M (1982b). Velocity of articulatory movements in normal and dysarthric subjects. Folia Phoniatrica 34: 210–15.

Hirose H, Kiritani S, Ushijima T, Sawashima M (1978). Analysis of abnormal articulatory dynamics in two dysarthric patients. Journal of Speech and Hearing Disorders 4: 96–105.

Hirose H, Kiritani S, Ushijima Y, Yoshioka H, Sawashima M (1981). Patterns of dysarthric movements in patients with parkinsonism. Folia Phoniatrica 33: 204–15.

Hirose H, Sawashima M, Niimi S (1985). Laryngeal dynamics in dysarthric speech. Paper presented at the Thirteenth World Congress of Otorhinolaryngology, Miami Beach.

Hoehn MM, Yahr MD (1967). Parkinsonism: onset, progression, and mortality. Neurology 17: 427–42.

Hoodin RB, Gilbert HR (1989a). Nasal airflows in parkinsonian speakers. Journal of Communication Disorders 22: 169–80.

Hoodin B, Gilbert HR (1989b). Parkinsonian dysarthria: an aerodynamic and perceptual description of velopharyngeal closure for speech. Folia Phoniatrica 41: 249–58.

Hovestadt A, Bogaard JD, Meerwaldt JD, van der Meche FGA, Stigt J (1989). Pulmonary function in Parkinson's disease. Journal of Neurology, Neurosurgery, and Psychiatry 42: 329–33.

Hunker C, Abbs JH, Barlow S (1982). The relationship between parkinsonian rigidity and hypokinesia in the orofacial system: a quantitative analysis. Neurology 32: 755–61.

Johnson JA, Pring TR (1990). Speech therapy and Parkinson's disease: a review and further data. British Journal of Disorders of Communiation 25: 183–94.

Kearns KP, Simons NN (1990). The efficacy of speech-language pathology intervention: motor speech disorders. Seminars in Speech and Language 11: 273–95.

Kent R, Netsell R (1975). A case study of an ataxic dysarthric: cineradiographic and spectrographic. Journal of Speech and Hearing Disorders 40: 115–34.

Kent R, Netsell R, Abbs JH (1979). Acoustic characteristics of dysarthria associated with cerebellar disease. Journal of Speech and Hearing Disorders 22: 613–26.

King JB, Ramig LO, Lemke JH, Horii Y (1994). Parkinson's disease: longitudinal changes in acoustic parameters of phonation. Journal of Medical Speech-Language Pathology 2: 29–42.

Kluin JJ, Gilman S, Markel DS, Koeppe RA, Rosenthal G, Junck L (1988). Speech disorders in olivopontocerebellar atrophy correlate with positron emission tomography findings. Annals of Neuorlogy 23: 547–54.

Laszewski Z (1956). Role of the Department of Rehabilitation in preoperative evaluation of Parkinsonian patients. Journal of the American Geriatric Society 4: 1280–4.

Lethlean JB, Chenery HJ, Murdoch BE (1990). Disturbed respiratory and prosodic function in Parkinson's disease: a perceptual and instrumental analysis. Australian Journal of Human Communication Disorders 18: 83–98.

Logemann JA, Fisher HB (1981). Vocal tract control in Parkinson's disease: phonetic feature analysis of misarticulations. Journal of Speech and Hearing Disorders 46: 348–52.

Logemann JA, Fisher HB, Boshes B, Blonsky ER (1978). Frequency and co-occurrence of vocal tract dysfunctions in the speech of a large sample of Parkinson's patients. Journal of Speech and Hearing Disorders 43: 47–57.

Ludlow CL, Bassich CJ (1983). The results of acoustic and perceptual assessment of two types of dysarthria. In Berry WR (ed.) Clinical Dysarthria. San Diego, CA: College Hill Press, pp.121–47.

Ludlow CL, Bassich CJ (1984). Relationships between perceptual ratings and acoustic measures of hypokinetic speech. In McNeil MR, Rosenbek JC, Aronson AE (eds) The Dysarthrias: Physiology, Acoustics, Perception, Management. San Diego, CA: College Hill Press, pp.163–95.

Martin JP (1968). Wilson's disease. In Vinken PJ, Bruyn GW (eds) Handbook of Clinical Neurology, Volume 6.. Amsterdam: North Holland, pp.267–78.

McClean MD, Beukelman DR, Yorkston KM (1987). Speech-muscle visuomotor tracking in dysarthric and nonimpaired speakers. Journal of Speech and Hearing Research 30: 276–82.

McNeil MR, Weismer G, Adams S, Mulligan M (1990). Oral structure nonspeech motor control in normal, dysarthric, aphasic, and apraxic speakers: isometric force and static position. Journal of Speech and Hearing Research 33: 255–68.

Metter EJ, Hanson WR (1986). Clinical and acoustical variability in hypokinetic dysarthria. Journal of Communication Disorders 19: 347–66.

Moore CA, Scudder RH (1989). Co-ordination of jaw muscle activity in parkinsonian movement: description and response to traditional treatment. In Yorkston KM, Beukelman DR (eds) Recent Advances in Clinical Dysarthria. Boston, MA: College Hill Press, pp.147–63.

Mueller PB (1971). Parkinson's disease: motor speech behaviour in a selected group of patients. Folia Phoniatrica 23: 333–46.

Murdoch BE (1990). Acquired Speech and Language Disorders: A Neuroanatomical and Functional Neurological Approach. London: Chapman and Hall.

Murdoch BE, Chenery JJ, Bowler S, Ingram JCL (1989). Respiratory function in Parkinson's subjects exhibiting a perceptible speech deficit: a kinematic and spirometric analysis. Journal of Speech and Hearing Disorders 54: 610–26.

Murdoch BE, Chenery JJ, Stokes PD, Hardcastle WJ (1991). Respiratory kinematics in speakers with cerebellar disease. Journal of Speech and Hearing Research 34: 768–80.

Murdoch BE, Manning CY, Theodoros DG, Thompson EC (1995). Laryngeal function in hypokinetic dysarthria. Paper presented at the XXIII World Congress of the International Association of Logopedics and Phoniatrics, Cairo, Egypt.

Murdoch G, Noble J, Chenery H, Ingram J (1989). A spirometric and kinematic analysis of respiratory function in pseudobulbar palsy. Australian Journal of Human Communication Disorders 17(2): 21–35.

Murdoch BE, Thompson EC, Stokes PD (1994). Phonatory and laryngeal dysfunction following upper motor neurone vascular lesions. Journal of Medical Speech-Language Pathology 2(3): 177–89.

Netsell R (1986). A Neurobiologic View of Speech Production and the Dysarthrias. San Diego, CA: College Hill.

Netsell R, Daniel B (1979). Dysarthria in adults: physiologic approach in rehabilitation. Archives of Physical Medicine and Rehabilitation 60: 502–8.

Netsell R, Daniel B, Celesia GG (1975). Acceleration and weakness in parkinsonian dysarthria. Journal of Speech and Hearing Disorders 40: 170–8.

Netsell R, Kent R (1976). Paroxysmal ataxic dysarthria. Journal of Speech and Hearing Disorders 41: 93–109.

Netsell R, Lotz WK, Barlow S (1989). A speech physiology examination for individuals with dysarthria. In Yorkston KM, Beukelman DR (eds) Recent Advances in Clinical Dysarthria. Boston, MA: College-Hill Press, pp.4–37.

Oder W, Grimm G, Kollegger H, Ferenci P, Schneider B, Deecke L (1991). Neurological and neuropsychiatric spectrum of Wilson's disease: a prospective study of 45 cases. Journal of Neurology 238: 281–7.

Oxtoby M (1982). Parkinson's Disease Patients and their Social Needs. London: Parkinson's Disease Society.

Ramig LO, Bonitati CM, Lemke JH, Horii Y (1994). Voice treatment for patients with Parkinson disease: development of an approach and preliminary efficacy data. Journal of Medical Speech-Language Pathology 2: 191–209.

Robbins J (1987). Swallowing in ALS and motor neuron disorders. Neurologic Clinics 5: 213–29.

Robbins JA, Logemann JA, Kirshner HS (1986). Swallowing and speech production in Parkinson's disease. Annals Neurology 19: 283–7.

Rosenbek JC, LaPointe LL (1978). The dysarthrias: description, diagnosis and treatment. In Johns DF (ed.) Clinical Management of Neurogenic Communication Disorders. Boston, MA: Little Brown, pp.251–310.

Rowland LP (1980). Motor neuron diseases: the clinical syndromes. In Mulder DW (ed.) The Diagnosis and Treatment of Amyotrophic Lateral Sclerosis. Boston, MA: Houghton Mifflin Professional Publishers, pp.7–27.

Sadiq SA, Thomas FP, Kilidireas K, Monroe A, Williams KP, Johnson D (1990). The spectrum of neurologic disease associated with anti-GM1 antibodies. Neurology 40: 1067–72.

Scott S, Caird FI (1983). Speech therapy for parkinson's disease. Journal of Neurology, Neurosurgery, and Psychiatry 46: 140–4.

Scott S, Caird FI, Williams BO (1985). Communication in Parkinson's Disease. London: Croom Helm.

Selby G (1968). Parkinson's Disease. In Vinken PJ, Bruyn GW (eds) Handbook of Clinical Neurology: Volume 6. Diseases of the Basal Ganglia. Amsterdam: North Holland, pp.173–211.

Solomon NP, Hixon TJ (1993). Speech breathing in Parkinson's disease. Journal of Speech and Hearing Research 36: 294–310.

Specola N, Vanier MT, Goutieres F, Mikol J, Aicardi J (1990). The juvenile and chronic forms of GM2 gangliosidosis: clinical and enzymatic heterogeneity. Neurology 40: 145–50.

Stacy M, Jankovic J (1993). Current approaches in the treatment of Parkinson's disease. Annual Review of Medicine 44: 431–40.

Starosta-Rubenstein S, Young AB, Kluin K, Hill G, Aisen AM, Gabrielsen T, Brewer GJ (1987). Clinical assessment of 31 patients with Wilson's disease. Archives of Neurology 44: 365–70.

Steele JC, Richardson JC, Olszewski J (1964). Progressive supra-nuclear palsy. Archives of Neurology 10: 333.

Streifler M, Hofman S (1984). Disorders of verbal expression Parkinsonism. Advances in Neurology 40: 385–93.

Stremmel W, Meyerrose K, Niederau C, Hefter H, Kreuzpaintner G, Strohmeyer G (1991). Wilson disease: clinical presentation, treatment, and survival. Annals of Internal Medicine 115: 720–6.

Svensson P, Henningson C, Karlsson S (1993). Speech motor control in Parkinson's disease: a comparison between a clinical assessment protocol and a quantitative analysis of mandibular movements. Folia Phoniatrica 45: 157–64.

Tandan R (1994). Clinical features and differential diagnosis of classical motor neuron disease. In Williams AC (ed.) Motor Neuron Disease. London: Chapman and Hall, pp.3–27.

Theodoros DG, Murdoch BE, Thompson EC (1995). Hypernasality in Parkinson's disease: a perceptual and physiological analysis. Journal of Medical Speech-Language Pathology 3: 73–84.

Thompson EC (1995). The physiological approach to dysarthria assessment and treatment: an examination in upper motor neurone dysarthria. Unpublished doctoral thesis. The University of Queenlsand, Australia.

Thompson EC, Murdoch BE (1995a). Interpreting the physiological bases of dysarthria from perceptual analyses: an examination of subjects with UMN type dysarthria. Australian Journal of Human Communication Disorders 23: 1–23.

Thompson EC, Murdoch BE (1995b). Disorders of nasality in subjects with upper motor neurone type dysarthria following cerebrovascular accident. Journal of Communication Disorders 28: 261–76.

Thompson EC, Murdoch BE, Stokes PD (1995a). Tongue function in subjects with upper motor neuron type dysarthria following cerebrovascular accident. Journal of Medical Speech-Language Pathology 3(1): 27–40.

Thompson EC, Murdoch BE, Stokes PD (1995b). Lip function in subjects with upper motor neurone type dysarthria following cerebrovascular accident. European Journal of Disorders of Communication 30: 451–66.

Thompson-Ward EC, Murdoch BE (1998). Instrumental assessment of the speech mechanism. In Murdoch BE (ed.) Dysarthria: A Physiological Approach to Assessment and Treatment. Cheltenham: Stanley Thornes, pp.68–101.

Uitti RJ, Calne DB (1993). Pathogenesis of idiopathic parkinsonism. European Neurology 33(Supplement 1): 6–23.

Van Oosten BW, Truyen L, Barkhof F, Polman CH (1995). Multiple sclerosis therapy. Drugs 49: 200–12.

Weismer G (1984). Acoustic descriptions of dysarthic speech: perceptual correlates and physiological inferences. Seminars in Speech and Language 5: 293–313.

Ziegler W, Von Cramon D (1986). Spastic dysarthria after acquired brain injury: an acoustic study. British Journal of Disorders of Communication 21: 173–87.

Zwirner P, Barnes GJ (1992). Vocal tract steadiness: a measure of phonatory and upper airway motor control during phonation in dysarthria. Journal of Speech and Hearing Research 35: 761–8.

Chapter 6
Dysarthria: an overview of treatment

KATHRYN M. YORKSTON and DAVID R. BEUKELMAN

Historians suggest that medical education can be characterized by a series of eras. The nineteenth century was the *era of diagnosis*, where new diseases and disorders were defined and characterized. The twentieth century was the *era of interventions*, where numerous methods for assessment and treatment were developed. The twenty-first century is predicted to be the *era of decision-making*, where medical education will be challenged to offer practitioners a structure by which decisions can be made to select and sequence intervention procedures. This chapter will be organized into three sections. The first, covers issues of description and diagnosis of the dysarthrias within the Institute of Medicine's model of disablement. The second, called 'Treatment: dealing with the consequences of dysarthria', describes issues of management of the consequences of dysarthria across the parameters of disablement. The third section, called 'Staging of treatment', describes sequencing of intervention, with an emphasis on how to make clinical decisions about who to treat, how to treat them and when to offer treatment.

The model of disablement: definitions of dysarthria

Dysarthria is a motor speech disorder caused by disturbances in neuro-muscular control of components of the speech mechanism. Weakness, spasticity or incoordination of the muscles because of damage to the central or peripheral nervous system causes difficulty in executing the movements of speech. The characteristics of dysarthria vary considerably, depending on the nature, severity and course of underlying neuropathology. A wide variety of neurological conditions result in dysarthria. Among the most common are Parkinson's disease, motor neurone disease, movement disorders, stroke, traumatic brain injury and cerebral palsy. More complete descriptions of the various types of dysarthria can be found elsewhere (Duffy, 1995; McNeil, 1997; Yorkston et al.,1999).

The World Health Organization's model of disablement and health is a useful framework from which to organize the definition of dysarthria (Pope and Tarlov, 1991). This model provides a means of classifying the consequences associated with health conditions, and thus, it also provides a means of organizing assessment and treatment techniques. In this model of the processes of disablement/enablement, five parameters are described: (a) *pathophysiological alterations*, which occur at the cellular or physiological level; (b) *impairments*, which occur as loss of function at a subsystem level; (c) *functional limitations*, which are reductions in the ability to function at the level of the organism or person because of an impairment; (d) *disabilities* are reductions in performance in natural environments; and (e) *societal limitations*, which are changes in performance that reduce or alter one's societal roles. These parameters can be used to define dysarthria (see Table 6.1).

The model's five parameters can also be used to differentiate between the various dysarthrias. As is illustrated in Table 6.1, the consequences of dysarthria vary across neurological conditions. For example, dysarthria associated with amyotrophic lateral sclerosis (ALS) is caused by the progressive degeneration of upper and lower motor neurones (the pathophysiology), which in turn leads to weakness and/or spasticity of the musculature of respiration, phonation and supralaryngeal articulation (the impairment). The impairment in the subsystems of speech production results in mixed spastic/flaccid dysarthria, characterized by reduced intelligibility and rate of speech (the functional limitation). This altered speech signal in turn leads to the speaker's reduced communication effectiveness in real-life situations, such as talking on the telephone or calling to someone in another room (the disability). The reduced speech performance in work-related situations may have other consequences, for example, the need to retire prematurely (the societal limitation).

By contrast, Table 6.1 also contains a description of the consequence of dysarthria associated with traumatic brain injury (TBI). Because the pathophysiology of TBI dysarthria is different from that of ALS, the pattern of speech impairment and functional limitation will also be different from that typical of ALS dysarthria. Because dysarthria in TBI may also be associated with cognitive and behaviour problems, the pattern of disability and societal limitation will also be unique compared with other dysarthrias. The neurological conditions of ALS and TBI serve to illustrate that the model of disablement can be applied to a variety of dysarthrias including those associated with Parkinson's disease, cerebral palsy, Huntington's disease, stroke and so on. The pattern of consequences for each type of dysarthria will vary depending on the underlying neurological condition.

Table 6.1: A conceptual framework for description of the consequences of dysarthria in amyotrophic lateral sclerosis and traumatic brain injury (adapted from work initially developed by the Institute of Medicine and published in *Disability in America*, 1991)

	Pathophysiology	Impairment	Functional limitation	Disability	Societal limitation
Definition	Interruption or interference of normal physiological and developmental processes or structures	Loss and/or abnormality of cognitive, emotional, physiological or anatomical structure or function; including secondary losses and pain	Restriction or lack of ability to perform an action or activity as compared to pre-injury performance; results from impairment	Inability or limitation in performing socially defined activities and roles within a social and physical environment as a result of internal or external factors and their interplay	Restriction attributable to social policy or barriers (structural or attitudinal) which limits fulfilment of roles or denies access to services or opportunities
Level of deficit	Cells and tissues	Components of the speech production process, including respiration, phonation, velopharyngeal function and oral articulatory structures	Speech performance with full range, speed, strength and coordination	Speech performance in a physical and social context	Performance of roles by speakers in social context
Dysarthria in ALS	Degeneration of upper and lower motor neurones	Weakness and/or spasticity in the bulbar musculature	Mixed spastic flaccid type with decreased speech intelligibility and rate	Decreased ability to communicate with a spouse in a different room	Premature retirement
Dysarthria in TBI	Damage to neural cells in cortical and subcortical structures	Varies depending on the underlying neuropathology, may include ataxia, spasticity and weakness	Mixed type with decreased speech intelligibility an naturalness	Decreased ability to introduce new topics in a conversation	Inability to return to work or school

If one is to understand fully the consequences of dysarthria, all of the parameters of the model of disablement must be considered. This broad perspective is necessary because characteristics of one level will not necessarily predict or reflect other levels. In other words, there is not always a one-to-one relationship between the parameters. For example, an impairment does not always lead to a disability of a similar magnitude. The following scenarios reflect some of the possible relationships among the levels.

A moderate impairment leading to some functional limitations but no disability: A 75-year-old man with a 15-year history of Parkinson's disease has speech typical of hypokinetic dysarthria. Vocal loudness and articulatory precision is reduced, but these changes do not interfere with speech intelligibility. He and his wife live independently and report no important changes in their communication style or their social roles.

A mild impairment and functional limitation associated with a severe disability and societal limitation: A 35-year-old college lecturer was diagnosed with multiple sclerosis. His speech is typical of a mild mixed spastic-ataxic dysarthria and is characterized by harsh voice quality, a slow speaking rate and an 'excess and equal' prosodic pattern that makes his speech seem unnatural. Some of his students wrote on his quarterly teaching evaluations that 'he doesn't seem very bright'. During a period of relapse in the multiple sclerosis, his contract for teaching during the following year was not renewed.

A moderate impairment associated with a severe functional limitation but only a moderate disability in a sheltered environment: A 25-year-old woman experienced a traumatic brain injury and ataxic dysarthria 7 years earlier. Her impairment was moderate and characterized by respiratory incoordination, and poor control of laryngeal and supralarygneal structures. Habitually, her speech was not intelligible; however, within the context of highly structured treatment tasks, she was able to make herself understood. She had difficulty with memory and new learning and would frequently behave impulsively. Within her group home, a high level of partner support and structure allowed her to function adequately within this sheltered environment. Thus, she experienced a moderate disability in a sheltered context. However, she experienced a severe societal limitation in that she would not develop or maintain many of the social roles that would be expected for a young women without disability.

Thus, the model of disablement and health reinforces the notion that the disability is not inherent in the individual, but rather is a product of the individual functioning within an environment (Brandt and Pope, 1997). The definitions provided by this model allow clinicians to consider intervention goals that not only focus on the individual but also on his or her social context.

Treatment: dealing with the consequences of dysarthria

For speech-language pathologists, dealing with the consequences of dysarthria means assessing contributors to the problem and devising treatment approaches that target important consequences. Intervention is typically focused on three of the five parameters of the model of disablement: impairment, functional limitation and disability. Table 6.2 illustrates examples of assessment and treatment activities in ALS and TBI. Note that both assessment and treatment may focus on multiple parameters simultaneously. For example, with dysarthria associated with TBI the treatment plan might include exercises to increase respiratory support for speech, training focusing on the use of the optimal speaking rate, and treatment that focuses on conversational interactions.

Treatment of the pathology

Typically, the medical community focuses on treatment of the pathology through a range of interventions, for example surgery or pharmacology. Although speech-language pathologists may be involved in measuring the outcomes of such interventions, they are not primarily responsible for decision-making at this level.

Treatment of the impairment

At times, the focus of intervention is to identify the pattern of physiological impairment and to reduce that impairment, in other words, to develop physiological support for speech. Documentation of the effects of physiological intervention has been the major focus of treatment research in dysarthria (Yorkston, 1996). A number of detailed case reports are available and describe the benefits of this physiological focus in individuals with TBI and stroke (Netsell and Daniel, 1979; Simpson, Till and Goff, 1988; Workinger and Netsell, 1992; Coelho et al., 1994; McHenry, Wilson and Minton, 1994).

The physiological approach is particularly relevant when the course of the dysarthria is stable or improving. Physiological intervention can be viewed as a process of creating the physiological building blocks of speech. These blocks are the minimal physiological requirements to support intelligible speech. If they are not present (as is the case with severe dysarthria), then one must work to develop the physiological components of speech.

Establishing respiratory support for speech

The respiratory system provides the energy source for speech production. Because it influences many other aspects of speech, it is frequently the initial focus of physiological intervention. Failure to establish respiratory-phonatory support for speech may be an important factor

Table 6.2: A conceptual framework for intervention of ALS and TBI dysarthria (adapted from work initially developed by the Institute of Medicine and published in *Disability in America*, 1991)

	Pathophysiology	Impairment	Functional limitation	Disability	Societal limitation
Examples of assessment targets for ALS dysarthria	Function of the upper and lower motor neurones	Ability to generate adequate subglottal pressure, or lingual strength	Speech intelligibility and rate	Decreased ability to be understood in natural communication settings	Employer interview
Examples of treatment targets for ALS dysarthria	No current treatment	Energy conversation techniques to prevent respiratory fatigue	shortening phrase length, and heightening stress patterning	Appropriate distance between speaker and listener, and Partner signal when messages are not understood	Scaffolding to support work-related activities
Examples of assessment targets for TBI dysarthria	Neural imaging techniques	Determining the speaker's ability to sustain appropriate subglottal air pressure	Speech intelligibility and naturalness	Interviews with the speaker and communication partners	Interview with school administrators
Examples of treatment targets for TBI dysarthria	Early pharmacological intervention to prevent cell death and brain swelling	Exercises to increase respiratory support for speech	Training the individual to reduce speaking rate	Teaching the speaker with dysarthria to indicate new topics	Modification of the school's policy

preventing the return of intelligible natural speech and necessitating the long-term use of augmentative communication approaches for individuals with cerebral palsy, TBI and brainstem stroke. The impact of respiratory impairment on the performance of speakers with dysarthria is a complex phenomenon. Perceptual indicators of respiratory inadequacy include inability to initiate phonation, abnormal loudness alterations, and abnormal patterns in the timing of inhalation and exhalation. Breath patterning abnormalities are characterized by a deviation from the normal speech breathing pattern of a quick inhalation followed by a prolonged exhalation.

If respiratory impairment is suspected, then assessment will focus on estimating the adequacy of respiratory support (the speaker's ability to sustain adequate levels of subglottal air pressure) and the pattern of respiratory movements. By measuring oral air pressure during the stop phase of the voiceless plosive sounds (such as the /p/), the clinician can estimate the amount of subglottal air pressure a speaker is using (Netsell, Lotz and Barlow, 1989; McHenry, 1996). Clinically, the 'five-for-five' rule is helpful (Netsell and Hixon, 1978). This rule suggests that if an individual is able to sustain 5 cm of water pressure with a bleed in the system, which allows a limited escape of air that must be replaced to sustain air pressure for 5 seconds, then respiratory support should be adequate for speech. Respiratory support for speech can also be estimated by assessing the speaker's ability to produce sustained phonation.

Respiratory movement, changes in shape of the thorax and abdomen during speech, may also be disrupted in dysarthria. Speakers with reduced vital capacity may routinely need to inhale more deeply prior to speaking than non-impaired individuals. Other individuals may fail to inhale before speaking and may begin to speak at improper lung volume levels. Still other individuals, particularly those with ataxic dysarthria, may exhibit a strong but uncoordinated respiratory system. These speakers may attempt to compensate for phonatory, velopharyngeal and articulatory problems by inhaling to excessively high lung volume level. This results in speech that is excessively loud.

The overall treatment goal for patients with respiratory impairments is to achieve a consistent subglottal air pressure during speech. A variety of approaches can be found in the literature. Blowing techniques, in which the speaker is taught to blow into a pressure sensor which contains a leak tube allowing air to escape at a rate associated with normal phonation, have been described for individuals with severe dysarthria (Netsell and Daniel, 1979; Hixon, Hawley and Wilson, 1982). Postural adjustments and prosthetic assistance have been reported to be of assistance to individuals with severe motor impairment (Rosenbek and LaPointe, 1985). Although there is no 'perfect' respiratory shape for speakers with dysarthria, patterns of speech breathing are fatiguing or unnatural for a speaker and should be eliminated with training.

Laryngeal function

Phonatory dysfunction associated with an impairment of the laryngeal system is common in dysarthria. This dysfunction may range from a severe impairment associated with the inability to generate a sound source or voice during speech, to a mild impairment associated with a slightly abnormal voice quality or vocal stability. Clinical assessment of phonatory dysfunction is made largely on the basis of perceptual judgements. These include judgements of features such as pitch level, pitch breaks and harsh or breathy voice quality. Instrumental measures of laryngeal function such as airflow through the vocal folds during phonation and laryngeal resistance are also available (Smitheran and Hixon, 1981; Netsell, 1984; D'Antonio et al., 1987).

Treatment of laryngeal impairment can be viewed as a hierarchy, from techniques appropriate for severe impairment to those appropriate for mild involvement. Intervention at the most severe levels focuses on establishment of voluntary phonation. Generally, an attempt is made to move from reflexive activities such as laughing and coughing to more voluntary voice production (Yorkston et al., 1999). Reduced vocal loudness, common in speakers with dysarthria, may be addressed by training the speaker to generate greater levels of subglottal air pressure. As in the case of loudness modification, training of respiratory and phonatory aspects of speech often go hand in hand. When voice quality disorders are associated with hyperadduction of the vocal folds, traditional voice therapy techniques designed to reduce laryngeal hyperadduction and increase airflow through the glottis may be appropriate (Prator and Swift, 1984) .

Velopharyngeal function

Velopharyngeal dysfunction of speakers with dysarthria is extremely important because it distorts the production of vowel and consonant sounds, thus exaggerating the impairment of other aspects of speech production such as respiratory-phonatory function and oral articulation. The patterns of velopharyngeal dysfunction in dysarthria include abnormal timing of velar movements related to other articulatory movement, incomplete velopharyngeal contact and inconsistency of movement (Netsell et al., 1989). Perceptual indicators of velopharyngeal impairment include presence of hypernasality, occurrence of nasal emission during the production of consonants, and a disproportionate inability to produce pressure consonants. Instrumentally, velopharyngeal function has been assessed using aerodynamic measures of oral air pressure and volume velocity of airflow across the velopharyngeal port (Warren, 1992). Direct visualization of the velopharyngeal mechanism can be achieved using fibre-optic equipment.

The three general categories of treatment approaches for speakers with velopharyngeal impairment are behavioural, prosthetic and surgical intervention. Generally, behavioural approaches are considered for speakers with mild or moderate impairment. These individuals are taught to achieve adequate velopharyngeal closure by speaking at the appropriate rate and adequately monitoring their general articulatory precision (Liss, Kuehn and Hinkle, 1994). The most common prosthetic method of treating velopharyngeal dysfunction in dysarthria speakers involves fitting of a palatal lift. A lift consists of a retentive portion that covers the hard palate and fastens to the maxillary teeth by wires, and a lift portion that extends along the oral surface of the soft palate. Discussion of candidacy and timing of palatal lift fitting with a speaker with TBI can be found elsewhere (Yorkston et al., 1989; Yorkston and Beukelman, 1991). Surgical procedures for velopharyngeal management have been reported on occasion (Dworkin and Johns, 1980).

Oral articulation

Impairment in oral articulatory function is almost universal in speakers with dysarthria. The most prevalent articulatory error in dysarthria is distortion of vowels and consonants. Treatment of oral articulatory impairment have often included attempts to normalize function. For example, exercises for strengthening the oral structures have been used with speakers with muscle weakness. However, caution is warranted because weakness is not universally present in dysarthria. Other abuses of strengthening exercises including delaying of the other intervention approaches until strengthening is 'finished' and increasing the strength of certain muscles so that they overwhelm the efforts of others (Rosenbek and LaPointe, 1985). Strengthening exercises are also contraindicated in some conditions such as ALS, where muscles do not rebound normally after fatigue. Other treatment approaches emphasize compensation for the impairment. For example, contrastive production or intelligibility drills have been used to assist speakers to modify production to make the final speech end product sound distinctive, for example to make 'pat' sound different from 'bat' (Yorkston, Beukelman and and Bell, 1988). These approaches do not attempt to train the speaker to change specific movement patterns. Instead, general feedback about the adequacy of the production is given and the speaker is expected to make the modifications necessary to accomplish the changes. Articulation may also be improved by global interventions such as increasing loudness and slowing speaking rate (Dromey, Ramig and Johnson, 1995).

Treatment of the functional limitation

Improvement in functional communication is a major focus of intervention effort in dysarthria. When dysarthria is severe this may involve the use of augmentative communication approaches rather than natural speech. For speakers with moderate dysarthria, speech intelligibility may be improved using speaking rate control techniques. For speakers with mild dysarthria, the emphasis in treatment may be on improving the naturalness of speech production.

Augmentative communication

The philosophy of augmentative communication applications has changed considerably in recent years (Beukelman and Mirenda, 1998). The focus of intervention has shifted from providing a single, long-term communication system for those individuals with persistent, severe dysarthria, to providing a series of systems that meet short-term communication needs while continuing efforts to re-establish natural speech. Case examples of the transitions through many augmentative systems are available for both speakers who are recovering from TBI (Light, Beesley and Collier, 1988) and individuals with ALS (Yorkston, Miller and Strand, 1995). Long-term follow-up studies of individuals with TBI who were non-speaking on admission to rehabilitation are also available (Dongilli, Hakel and Beukelman, 1992; Ladtkow and Culp, 1992). These studies suggest that about half of these individuals become functional natural speakers during inpatient rehabilitation, often when they are no longer agitated.

Rate control

Rate reduction is an important strategy in speech treatment with speakers with dysarthria. Ataxia is a frequent component of dysarthria in a number of disability conditions including TBI, degenerative cerebellar disorders and multiple sclerosis. Sudden onset of ataxia, coupled with poor monitoring associated with reduced cognitive functioning, frequently contributes to unintelligible speech. A variety of rate control techniques are available (Yorkston et al., 1999). Some of these techniques are described as rigid because they impose a slow speaking rate, often at the expense of speech naturalness. Included in the category of rigid techniques are alphabet supplementation (where the speaker points to the first letter of each word as the word is spoken) and pacing boards (where the speaker points to a different location on a colour board as each word is spoken). These techniques are generally reserved for those speakers who cannot learn to speak more slowly using other techniques. Computerized rhythmic pacing (Beukelman, Yorkston and Tice, 1997) and delayed auditory feedback (Adams, 1994) are techniques that slow speaking rate but preserve speech naturalness.

Maximizing speech naturalness

For individuals with mild dysarthria, speech naturalness often remains a concern when speech intelligibility is good. To achieve natural-sounding speech, attention is focused on the prosodic or melodic components of speech including stress patterning, intonation and rhythm. Contributors to reduced naturalness of speech include monotony (an excessively even rhythmic patterning of syllables, an evenness of stress patterning or reduction in intonation contours), and mismatches between the prosodic features and the grammar of the utterance (Bellaire, Yorkston and Beukelman, 1986).

Treatment for the disability

Comprehensibility has been defined as the extent to which a listener understands utterances produced by a dysarthric speaker in a natural communication situation (Yorkston, Strand and Kennedy, 1996). The adequacy of communication can be improved by a variety of simple techniques (Vogel and Miller, 1991). For example, speakers with decreased speech intelligibility may improve the adequacy of communication by introducing a new topic in writing and by signalling to the listener when they are changing topics. Other techniques to improve comprehensibility involve the listener and the communication environment. Severely distorted speech is easier to understand if the room is quiet and listeners are able to watch the speaker's face. Intervention focusing on improved comprehensibility of speech is dependent on a detailed understanding of the environments in which communication is likely to occur and on well-instructed communication partners who take an active role in facilitating the communicative interaction.

Staging of treatment

Staging of the disease process is a model used by many fields of medicine as a tool in decision-making. Staging of intervention is the sequencing of management so that current problems are addressed and future problems anticipated. Staging is important in dysarthria intervention because many of the conditions associated with dysarthria are not stable. Individuals with acquired dysarthria associated with stroke or TBI experience a period of spontaneous recovery before their neurological condition stabilizes. Individuals with congenital conditions such as cerebral palsy progress through developmental stages. With advanced age, dysarthria in these individuals may become more severe. Finally, many conditions associated with dysarthria are progressive, including motor neurone disease, Parkinson's disease, Huntington's disease and others. Staging of intervention is based on knowledge of the disease process and the provision of intervention in an appropriate and timely fashion.

The staging system described in this chapter is based on the severity of functional limitation. Three clinical populations frequently associated with dysarthria were selected because of their varying clinical course: TBI with a stable or recovering course, Parkinson's disease with a slowly progressive course, and ALS with a rapidly progressive course. The staging system proposed here is chronological. For example, the staging of TBI begins with early severe functional limitations and proceeds through less severe limitations. On the other hand, staging in the degenerative diseases begins with early, mild limitations and proceeds to more severe limitations. At each stage, the relative importance of three general approaches to intervention will be reviewed: physiological approaches (those that focus on the impairment), functional approaches (those that focus on the functional limitation), and approaches based on social systems (those that focus on the disability and social limitations). The relative importance of these various approaches will vary from stage to stage and across populations.

Traumatic brain injury (TBI)

Dysarthria associated with TBI varies considerably both in type and severity. This section summarizes five stages of intervention for dysarthria in TBI. At each stage, the features of functional limitation in dysarthria will be described, along with some common speech and augmentative communication treatment approaches at the levels of speech physiology, functional limitation and social systems. Because the speakers' level of awareness and cognition play an important role in this intervention, issues related to cognitive function will also be described at each stage.

Stage 1 – no useful speech

This stage is characterized by the absence of useful speech. This may occur early after the injury and may be the result of a number of factors, including poor cognition or reduced arousal, severe motor deficits or severe language deficits. When severe motor impairment exists, speech intervention focuses on establishing the physiological support for speech. Typically, this involves work with the various speech subsystems in non-speech tasks. For example, blow-bottle tasks may be used to establish adequate respiratory support (Hixon et al., 1982). Focus is typically placed on basic respiratory/phonatory function because these systems are frequently major contributors to poor speech function.

Because of the severity of the dysarthria, physiological exercises must be supplemented by the development of augmentative communication approaches in order to establish functional communication. Three phases of intervention have been proposed as the sequence for establishing a basic augmentative communication system in individuals with TBI (Ladtkow and Culp, 1992). During the early period of recovery, augmentative communication approaches may involve the development of initial choice-making, such as establishing a consistent yes/no system. The next phase of augmentative communication may involve pointing to simple alphabet boards. If motor deficits do not resolve as the level of cognitive function improves, the final phase is the development of multiple purpose augmentative communication devices. Because augmentative communication approaches for severe dysarthria depend on the level of cognitive function, most are simple (DeRuyter and Lafontaine, 1987; DeRuyter and Kennedy, 1991). They may involve communication of basic needs and require a high level of environmental structure and partner support. These systems usually are based on direct selection of items rather than on complex coding for message retrieval.

Stage 2 – natural speech supplemented by augmentative communication

At this stage, natural speech can be used to carry part of the communicative load; however, communication is often easier if speech is supplemented with augmentative communication techniques. Exercises focusing on speech physiology move from predominately non-speech activities used in the early stages of dysarthria intervention to speech-like tasks. For example, once an individual is able to achieve minimal competencies, respiratory-phonatory exercises such as blow-bottles shift to more speech-like tasks such as sustained phonation or producing short phrases with good voicing. This stage of intervention can be viewed as a period of transition from dependence on simple augmentative systems to the use of natural speech. Alphabet supplementation and word boards are often used to introduce topics. Hustad and colleagues suggest that individuals with severe dysarthria may be taught to use expectation dictionaries (Hustad, Beukelman and Yorkston, 1998). These are lists of words or short phrases that speakers are actively practising in treatment. When attempting to understand these highly distorted messages, listeners are assisted by referring to the list of potential options.

Issues related to communication in social contexts must also be addressed at this stage. Depending on the level of cognitive function, communication partners may be taught to take more or less responsibility for managing the interaction. Thus, they may need to establish or confirm the topic of conversation, guide the resolution of communication breakdowns, or structure the communication environment so that noise is reduced.

Stage 3 – reduction in speech intelligibility

At this stage, natural speech may be the primary means of communication although dysarthria is obvious and may require modification of the communication environment. Speech exercises involve production of meaningful utterances rather than extensive use of non-speech or speech-like activities. For example, blow-bottle exercises (non-speech tasks) and sustained phonation exercises (speech-like activities) give way to exercises that teach speakers to initiate meaningful utterances at the appropriate lung volume level. Practice utterances are selected based on their importance and usefulness for the speaker. Treatment targets the specific aspects of speech that seem to be interfering with intelligibility. For example, if the speaker has not adopted the appropriate speaking rate, then treatment may focus on rate control. The focus of intervention is also on understanding the environments where communication takes place. Speakers with dysarthria may be taught to optimize their communication environment and manage their communication partners. Some speakers need assistance in doing this effectively. If this is the case, listeners may be trained to help structure the communicative exchange (Yorkston et al., 1996).

Stage 4 – obvious disorder with intelligible speech

Dysarthria may persist at this stage. Although speech intelligibility is not reduced, speech rate and naturalness are typically affected. Exercises to develop physiological support for speech are less important at this stage than they were at earlier stages. Thus, relatively little emphasis is placed on exercises that target the individual speech subsystem.

Naturalness, or lack of it, does not usually involve a single speech subsystem. Therefore, treatment usually focuses on some simple, overall aspect of speech that will have an impact on a variety of symptoms. For example, the speaker with dysarthria may be taught to heighten stress patterning or to produce 'clear speech'. Both of these techniques have global influences on speech production but require that the speaker attends to only one instruction at a time, thus simplifying the speaker's task. Depending on the speaker's cognitive status, they are taught to manage good speaking strategies in a variety of natural contexts. Treatment may shift from a focus on speech production to a focus on the pragmatic aspects of communication such as turn-taking, topic maintenance and so on (Gillis, 1996; Yorkston and Kennedy, 1999).

Stage 5 – no detectable motor speech disorder

Although individuals at this stage may not have a detectable motor speech disorder, they may still have considerable residual communication disorders that are reflected mostly in the areas of discourse and pragmatics. Treatment focusing on the physiological components of speech are generally not appropriate for speakers at this stage. However, speech production may still deserve some attention. Frequently, no problem with speech is evident if the speaker is asked to perform a very controlled set of tasks with few cognitive demands, but speech may call attention to itself in cognitively demanding situations. For example, intonation and pause structure may become more unusual if the speaker is communicating novel information or presenting an argument as part of a public presentation. Therefore, intervention may focus on the areas of discourse and pragmatics and the use of 'good speech' in complex communication situations.

Parkinson's disease

The severity of the hypokinetic dysarthria associated with Parkinson's disease may vary from absence, through mild and moderate, to severe. Because the focus of intervention, at least in part, depends on the severity of the functional limitation, the stages of intervention are summarized in the following section. In each stage, the features of the speech will be described, along with some common treatment approaches.

Stage 1 – no detectable speech disorder

This is the stage when the diagnosis of Parkinson's disease has been made. Because speech symptoms are typically not present in early stages of the disease, treatment focusing on physiological exercises is typically not indicated. On the other hand, preventive exercises that focus on enhanced speech production may be considered for those with Parkinson's disease who engage in highly demanding communication activities. For example, lecturers or ministers may benefit from intervention that focuses on maintaining their superior public speaking skills. These activities may involve producing speech that is loud, clear and expressive. During this stage of intervention, individuals with Parkinson's disease and their family members may also engage in educational activities. Because of the decreased sensitivity to the magnitude of their symptoms, some speakers may need to seek the feedback of others closely associated with them to monitor the appearance of mild symptoms.

Stage 2 – obvious speech disorder with intelligible speech

At this stage, changes in the voice are typically the first speech features to be observed in individuals with Parkinson's disease. These symptoms include reduced loudness, monotony and breathiness. Treatment approaches at this stage include techniques that focus on the physiological aspects of speech production. For example, speakers with Parkinson's disease may be taught a series of exercises designed to increase vocal fold adduction, to maximize duration of phonation, and to increase respiratory support. These exercises involve practising to improved loudness in increasingly difficult speech activities (Ramig, Pawlas and Countryman, 1995; Ramig et al., 1996). Attention to the practice of good speech habits in natural communication situations is also warranted. Individuals with Parkinson's disease often have difficulty scaling the size of their movements. This may lead to a general reduction in the extent of articulatory movements. Therefore, focus is also placed on increasing the self-perceived level of effort that is expended during speech production. As with all stages of dysarthria associated with Parkinson's disease, client and family education is a critical part of intervention.

Stage 3 – reduction in speech intelligibility

A reduction in speech intelligibility in certain situations is a key feature distinguishing this stage from the previous one. Both voice and articulation are abnormal. Focus on increasing respiratory-phonatory effort may take the form of asking speakers to produce increasing longer-sustained phonation and then move the new louder voice into production of speech utterance (Ramig, Pawlas and Countryman, 1995). A variety of techniques may be effective in slowing speaker rate. Speakers may be taught to consider speech as a 'performance' where they are no longer regular speakers but where they imagine themselves to be public speakers or performers (Sullivan, Brune and Beukelman, 1996). There is a continuing need to encourage speakers to use a high level of effort. A group treatment setting may be appropriate so that speakers can learn to appreciate feedback from listeners regarding their overall speech adequacy (Sullivan et al., 1996). Videotaping of speech performance may also serve as a useful tool to provide feedback to the speaker.

Stage 4 – natural speech supplemented by augmentative techniques

At this stage, natural speech alone is no longer a functional means of communication. This is usually the consequence of a reduced ability to initiate speech movements, decreased vocal loudness, and limited articulatory movements. Exercises focusing on the physiological subsystems of speech may be of limited benefit at this stage because of difficulty with new motor learning. Treatment may focus on the supplementation of natural speech with augmentative communication approaches such as alphabet supplementation or use of delayed auditory feedback devices (Adams, 1997). Listeners must take considerable responsibility in using augmentative communication techniques and in the resolution of communication breakdowns.

Stage 5 – no functional speech

A small percentage of individuals in the advanced stage of Parkinson's disease lose all functional speech. Physiological exercises are typically of little benefit at this stage. Given the overall motor control impairment associated with Parkinson's disease, which is frequently complicated by cognitive impairment, complex augmentative communication intervention is difficult to institute and must be individualized. Listeners must take most of the responsibility for maintaining communication interactions.

Amyotrophic lateral sclerosis (ALS)

Dysarthria associated with ALS may be an initial symptom in the bulbar form of the disease. As the disease progresses, a pattern of mixed spastic, flaccid dysarthria emerges. Profound weakness and spasticity may occur relatively rapidly, thus necessitating the use of augmentative communication devices for some individuals (Yorkston et al., 1993). Linguistic or cognitive changes are typically not limiting factors. The staging of intervention is summarized in the following section.

Stage 1 – no detectable speech disorder

Because no speech changes are detectable at this stage, physiological exercises are typically not indicated. Unlike speakers with Parkinson's disease, who may be unaware of changing speech, speakers with ALS are typically keenly aware of speech changes. Some speakers may notice a change in the effort needed during demanding speaking activities such as public speaking. In addition to confirming the normalcy of speech, techniques for energy conservation may be warranted. Information about the natural course of the communication changes typically associated with ALS is frequently requested. Therefore, it is important for clients to know that services and assistance are available when they are needed and that these services will allow maintenance of functional speech.

Stage 2 – obvious speech disorder with intelligible speech

At this stage, both the speaker and frequent communication partners notice changes in speech. These changes may become more pronounced with fatigue. Energy conversation techniques are important. These may include some modification in speaking patterns to ensure that individuals with ALS are speaking at an appropriate lung volume level. Speakers are cautioned against exercising to the point of fatigue. Most individuals with ALS begin to reduce their speaking rates to minimize the speech disturbance and maintain speech intelligibility. The need for slowed speaking rates should be explained and encouraged. Intervention focusing on natural communication contexts may include minimizing environmental adversity, establishing the context of the message, encouraging communication partners with hearing loss to use aids and teaching strategies for coping with communication in groups (Yorkston, Miller and Strand, 1995).

Stage 3 – reduction in speech intelligibility

At this stage, changes in speaking rate, articulation and resonance are all evident. Intervention activities that require a great deal of exercise and repetition of movement at maximum effort levels should be avoided because individuals with ALS may not rebound from muscular fatigue as others would. Non-fatiguing exercises to maintain range of motion and reducing laryngeal spasticity may be helpful. Speakers may need to exaggerate articulatory movements. Speakers at this stage may also need to repeat their messages when they are not understood. Partners become more active in breakdown resolution strategies or play the role of translator for the speaker with ALS.

Stage 4 – natural speech supplemented by augmentative techniques

At this stage, natural speech alone is no longer a functional means of communication. Physiological exercises are typically not indicated. Intervention for speakers at this stage may include alphabet supplementation, changing communication modes for different message types (greeting versus new information) and different communication partners, alerting systems, augmented telephone communication and portable writing systems.

Stage 5 – no functional speech

Speakers with advanced bulbar ALS have lost functional speech. Intervention for speakers at this stage may include establishing a reliable yes/no system, handwriting, eye-gaze systems, and communication systems for speakers dependent on ventilators. Augmentative communication systems are used to support communication on the telephone, with strangers, for detailed written messages, and on the internet (Beukelman, Mathy and Yorkston, 1998).

The staging of functional limitation in dysarthria has the potential to assist in making clinical decisions about how to treat speakers with dysarthria and when to apply various types of intervention. It can be viewed as an important part of outcomes measurement because it provides a means of describing the process of intervention. Frattali writes '. . . process and outcome are fundamentally linked in a single, symmetrical structure that makes of one almost a mirror image of the other' (Frattali, 1998: 4). She further states (p.176): 'Quality of clinical care can be improved only if its processes are understood, defined, and employed consistently and appropriately to reduce their variances and the unpredictability of the outcome.'

Treatment efficacy

In contrast to traditional medical models where intervention is judged as successful if symptoms of disease are alleviated, functional models of rehabilitation view success as 'restoration of function' (Granger and Fiedler, 1997). In clinical practice, the model of disablement has provided a basis on which a variety of decisions about treatment efficacy can be based. The model suggests that multiple levels of assessment are needed. For speakers with stable or improving pathology and impairment, measures of functional limitation such as speech intelligibility and naturalness are important indicators of outcome, and thus the effectiveness of treatment. For speakers with degenerative diseases, outcome assessment is complicated because the speech impairment will not improve. However, when taught appropriate compensatory or supplementary communication strategies, measures of functional communication may stabilize or even improve, and thus the benefits of treatment can be documented.

Because of increasing scrutiny of healthcare costs, documentation of the effectiveness of intervention approaches has been given new priority: 'We do not know nearly as much about the effectiveness of treatment as we should' (Duffy, 1995: 386). The field of dysarthria is not unique in this lack of evidence. Somewhat surprisingly, most medical services are not supported by strong, data-based evidence or expert opinion. The Institute of Medicine guidelines committee estimated that for 4% of all health services, the scientific evidence is strong; for about 45% of patient care, evidence is modest; and for another 51% the evidence is very sparse or non-existent (Institute of Medicine, 1992).

Recently, the field of motor speech disorders has seen an increase in publications related to treatment efficacy and intervention outcomes (Yorkston, 1996; Hustad et al., 1998). Generally, three types of question are addressed in the efficacy literature: does treatment work? does one treatment work better than another? and, in what ways does treatment alter behaviour (Olswang, 1990)? Some of the treatment efficacy literature in the field of dysarthria focuses on general approaches to intervention with specific populations, such as individuals with ALS or Parkinson's disease (Yorkston et al., 1993; Ramig et al., 1995). Perhaps the most ambitious of the recent treatment studies is the one conducted by Ramig and her colleagues (Ramig et al., 1994). In this study, 40 individuals with idiopathic Parkinson's disease underwent a four-week intervention programme aimed at increasing phonatory effort. A variety of acoustic and perceptual measures showed post-treatment improvement and maintenance of that improvement at six- and 12-month follow-up. Because of the progressive nature of their disorder, maintenance of treatment effects is particularly encouraging in this group study of the parkinsonian population.

Other literature provides reviews of specific techniques including EMG biofeedback (Gentil et al., 1994), training the velopharyngeal musculature (Liss et al., 1994), and effects of speaker instruction (Hammen and Yorkston, 1994; Kennedy, Strand and Yorkston, 1994). Because the type of dysarthria is important in selecting specific treatment approaches, Duffy (1995: 404–10) provides a summary of treatment approaches that may be beneficial for various dysarthria types. Possibly because dysarthric speakers differ so much from one another and thus require individual interventions, most of the treatment studies are case reports. A variety of treatment approaches have been reported in case studies including delayed auditory feedback (Adams, 1994), continuous positive airway pressure (CPAP) (Kuehn and Wachtel, 1994), palatal lift prosthesis (McHenry et al., 1994), increasing phonatory effort (Countryman, Ramig and Pawlas, 1994), and behavioural training (Hodge and Hall, 1994). Because reports of treatment efficacy are typically based on research literature and are usually limited to published reports, gaps in the evidence are apparent. It is hoped that these gaps will be bridged as clinical researchers continue to make advances in the measurement and treatment of individuals with dysarthria.

Summary

In this chapter, dysarthria has been viewed from the perspective of the model of disablement. This model provides a useful schema for organizing the consequences of chronic diseases such as stroke, Parkinson's disease or ALS and other conditions. Using this model, dysarthria is defined as an impairment involving the components of the speech production mechanism including the respiratory, phonatory, velopharyngeal and oral articulatory systems. Because of this impairment, speech function may be altered in rate, intelligibility and naturalness. The altered speech function in turn may lead to reduced speech effectiveness in natural communication contexts. Comprehensive assessment and intervention for speakers with dysarthria result in an understanding of all of the levels of the disablement process. Finally, intervention also involves the staging of treatment in which sequences of intervention approaches are selected. These sequences will differ depending on the underlying neuropathology and on the natural course of the dysarthria, and may be based on the severity of functional limitations. The appropriate sequence of intervention responds to present needs and anticipates future problems for speakers with dysarthria and their communication partners.

Acknowledgement

The preparation of this chapter was supported in part by the Barkley Trust.

References

Adams SG (1994). Accelerating speech in a case of hypokinetic dysarthria: descriptions and treatment. In Till JA, Yorkston KM, Beukelman DR (eds) Motor Speech Disorders: Advances in Assessment and Treatment. Baltimore, MD: Paul H. Brookes, pp.213–28.

Adams SG (1997). Hypokinetic dysarthria in Parkinson's disease. In McNeil MR (ed.) Clinical Management of Sensorimotor Speech Disorders. New York: Thieme, pp.261–86.

Bellaire K, Yorkston KM, Beukelman DR (1986). Modification of breath patterning to increase naturalness of a mildly dysarthric speaker. Journal of Communication Disorders 19: 271–80.

Beukelman DR, Mathy P, Yorkston KM (1998). Outcomes measurements of motor speech disorders. In Frattali C (ed.) Measuring Outcomes in Speech-language Pathology. New York: Thieme, pp.334–53.

Beukelman DR, Mirenda P (1998). Augmentative and Alternative Communication: Management of Severe Communication Disorders in Children and Adults (2nd edition). Baltimore, MD: Paul H. Brookes.

Beukelman DR, Yorkston KM, Tice R (1997). Pacer/tally Rate Measurement Software. Lincoln, NE: Tice Technology Services.

Brandt EN, Pope AM (eds) (1997). Enabling America: Assessing the Role of Rehabilitation Science and Engineering. Washington, DC: National Academy Press.

Coelho CA, Gracco VL, Fourakis M, Rossetti M, Oshima K (1994). Application of instrumental techniques in the assessment of dysarthria: a case study. In Till JA, Yorkston KM, Beukelman DR (eds) Motor Speech Disorders: Advances in Assessment and Treatment. Baltimore, MD: Paul H. Brooke, pp.103–18.

Countryman S, Ramig LO, Pawlas AA (1994). Speech and voice deficits in parkinsonism plus syndromes: can they be treated? Journal of Medical Speech-Language Pathology 2(3): 211–26.

D'Antonio L, Chait D, Lotz W, Netsell R (1987). Perceptual-physiologic approach to evaluation and treatment of dysphonia. Annals of Otology, Rhinology and Laryngology 2: 182–90.

DeRuyter F, Kennedy MR (1991). Augmentative communication following traumatic brain injury. In Beukelman DR, Yorkston KM (eds) Communication Disorders following Traumatic Brain Injury: Management of Cognitive, Language, and Motor Impairments. Austin, TX: ProEd, pp.317–65.

DeRuyter F, Lafontaine LM (1987). The nonspeaking brain injured: a clinical and demographic database report. Augmentative and Alternative Communication 3: 18–25.

Dongilli JP, Hakel M, Beukelman D (1992). Recovery of functional speech following traumatic brain injury. Journal of Head Trauma Rehabilitation 7: 91–101.

Dromey C, Ramig LO, Johnson AB (1995). Phonatory and articulatory changes associated with increased vocal intensity in Parkinson disease: a case study. Journal of Speech & Hearing Research 38(4): 751–64.

Duffy JR (1995). Motor Speech Disorders: Substrates, Differential Diagnosis, and Management. St Louis, MO: Mosby.

Dworkin JR, Johns DF (1980). Management of velopharyngeal incompetence in dysarthria: a historical review. Clinical Otolaryngology 5: 61.

Frattali C (1998). Measuring Outcomes in Speech-language Pathology. New York: Thieme.

Gentil M, Aucouturier JL, Delong V, Sambuis E (1994). EMG biofeedback in the treatment of dysarthria. Folia Phoniatrica et Logopedica 46(4): 188–92.

Gillis RJ (1996). Traumatic Brain Injury Rehabilitation for Speech-language Pathologists. Boston, MA: Butterworth-Heinemann.

Granger CV, Fiedler RC (1997). The measurement of disability. In Fuhrer M (ed.) Assessing Medical Rehabilitation Practices. Baltimore, MD: Paul H. Brookes, pp.103–23.

Hammen VL, Yorkston KM (1994). Effect of instruction on selected aerodynamic parameters in subjects with dysarthria and control subjects. In Till JA, Yorkston KM, Beukelman DR (eds) Motor Speech Disorders: Advances in Assessment and Treatment. Baltimore, MD: Paul H. Brookes, pp.161–74.

Hixon T, Hawley J, Wilson J (1982). An around-the-house device for the clinical determination of respiratory driving pressure. Journal of Speech & Hearing Disorders 47: 413–15.

Hustad KC, Beukelman DR, Yorkston KM (1998). Functional outcome assessment in dysarthria. Seminars in Speech & Language 19: 289–300.

Institute of Medicine (1991) Disability in America: Toward a national agenda for prevention. Washington DC: National Academy Press.

Institute of Medicine (1992). Guidelines for clinical practice: from development to use, edited by MJ Field and KN Lohr. Washington, DC: National Academy Press.

Kennedy MRT, Strand EA, Yorkston KM (1994). Selected acoustic changes in the verbal repairs of dysarthric speakers. Journal of Medical Speech-Language Pathology 2(4): 263–80.

Kuehn DP, Wachtel JM (1994). CPAP therapy for treating hypernasality following closed head injury. In Till JA, Yorkston KM, Beukelman DR (eds) Motor Speech Disorders: Advances in Assessment and Treatment. Baltimore, MD: Paul H. Brookes, pp.207–12.

Ladtkow MC, Culp D (1992). Augmentative communication with the traumatic brain-injured population. In Yorkston KM (ed.) Augmentative Communication in the Medical Setting. Tucson, AZ: Communication Skill Builders, pp.139–244.

Light J, Beesley M, Collier B (1988). Transition through multiple augmentative and alternative communication systems: a three-year case study of a head injury adolescent. Augmentative & Alternative Communication 4: 2–14.

Liss JM, Kuehn DP, Hinkle KP (1994). Direct training of velopharyngeal musculature. Journal of Medical Speech-Language Pathology 2(3): 243–51.

McHenry M (1996). Motor speech disorders. In Gillis RJ (ed.) Traumatic Brain Injury: Rehabilitation for Speech-language Pathologists. Boston, MA: Butterworth-Heinemann, pp.223–54.

McHenry MA, Wilson RL, Minton JT (1994). Management of multiple physiological deficits following traumatic brain injury. Journal of Medical Speech-Language Pathology 2: 58–74.

McNeil MR (ed.) (1997). Clinical Management of Sensorimotor Speech Disorders. New York: Thieme.

Netsell R (1984). Physiological studies of dysarthria and their relevance to treatment. Seminars in Language 5(4): 279–92.

Netsell R, Daniel B (1979). Dysarthria in adults: physiologic approach to rehabilitation. Archives of Physical Medicine and Rehabilitation 60: 502.

Netsell R, Hixon T (1978). A noninvasive method for clinically estimating subglottal air pressure. Journal of Speech and Hearing Disorders 43: 326–30.

Netsell R, Lotz WK, Barlow SM (1989). A speech physiology examination for individuals with dysarthria. In Yorkston KM, Beukelman DR (eds) Recent Advances in Clinical Dysarthria. Boston, MA: College-Hill Press, pp.3–33.

Olswang LB (1990). Treatment efficacy: the breadth of research. In Olswang LB, Thompson CK, Warren SF, Minghetti NJ (eds) Treatment Efficacy Research in Communication Disorders. Rockville, MD: American Speech-Language-Hearing Foundation, pp.99–103.

Pope AM, Tarlov AR (eds) (1991). Disability in America: Toward a National Agenda for Prevention. Washington, DC: National Academy Press.

Prator RJ, Swift R (1984). Manual of Voice Therapy. Boston, MA: Little, Brown.

Ramig LO, Bonitati CM, Lemke JH, Horii Y (1994). Voice treatment for patients with Parkinson disease: development of an approach and preliminary efficacy data. Journal of Medical Speech-Language Pathology 2(3): 191–210.

Ramig LO, Countryman S, Thompson LL, Horii Y (1995). A comparison of two forms of intensive speech treatment in Parkinson disease. Journal of Speech & Hearing Research 38: 1232–51.

Ramig LO, Countryman S, O'Brien C, Hoehn M, Thompson L (1996). Intensive speech treatment for patients with Parkinson disease: short and long-term comparison of two techniques. Neurology 47: 1496–503.

Ramig LO, Pawlas AA, Countryman S (1995). The Lee Silverman Voice Treatment. Iowa City, IA: National Center for Voice and Speech.

Rosenbek JC, LaPointe LL (1985). The dysarthrias: description, diagnosis, and treatment. In Johns D (ed.) Clinical Management of Neurogenic Communication Disorders. Boston, MA: Little Brown, pp.97–152.

Simpson MB, Till JA, Goff AM (1988). Long-term treatment of severe dysarthria: a case study. Journal of Speech & Hearing Disorders 53: 433–40.

Smitheran J, Hixon T (1981). A clinical method for estimating laryngeal airway resistance during vowel production. Journal of Speech & Hearing Disorders 46: 138–46.

Sullivan MD, Brune PJ, Beukelman DR (1996). Maintenance of speech changes following group treatment for hypokinetic dysarthria of Parkinson's disease. In Robin DA, Yorkston KM, Beukelman DR (eds) Disorders of Motor Speech: Assessment, Treatment and Clinical Characterization. Baltimore, MD: Paul H. Brookes, pp.287–310.

Vogel D, Miller L (1991). A top-down approach to treatment of dysarthric speech. In Vogel D, Cannito M (eds) Treating Disordered Speech Motor Control. Austin, TX: Pro-Ed, pp.87–109.

Warren DW (1992). Aerodynamic measurement of speech. In Cooper J (ed.) Assessment of Speech and Voice Production: Research and Clinical Applications, NIDCD Monograph. Bethesda, MD: National Institute of Deafness and Other Communication Disorders, pp.103–11.

Workinger MS, Netsell R (1992). Restoration of intelligible speech 13 years post-head injury. Brain Injury 6(2): 183–7.

Yorkston KM (1996). Treatment efficacy: dysarthria. Journal of Speech & Hearing Research 39(5): S46–S57.

Yorkston KM, Beukelman DR (1991). Motor speech disorders. In Beukelman DR, Yorkston KM (eds) Communication Disorders Following Traumatic Brain Injury: Management of Cognitive, Language, and Motor Impairment. Boston, MA: College-Hill Press, pp.251–316.

Yorkston KM, Beukelman DR, Bell KR (1988). Clinical Management of Dysarthric Speakers. Austin, TX: Pro-Ed.

Yorkston KM, Beukelman DR, Strand EA, Bell KR (1999). Management of Motor Speech Disorders in Children and Adults. Austin, TX: Pro-Ed.

Yorkston KM, Honsinger MJ, Beukelman DR, Taylor T (1989). The effects of palatal lift fitting on the perceived articulatory adequacy of dysarthric speakers. In Yorkston KM, Beukelman DR (eds) Recent Advances in Clinical Dysarthria. Boston, MA: College-Hill Press, pp.85–98.

Yorkston KM, Kennedy MRT (1999). Treatment approaches for communication disorders. In Rosenthal M (ed.) Rehabilitation of the Adult and Child with Traumatic Brain Injury (2nd edition). Philadelphia, PA: FA Davis, pp. 284–96.

Yorkston KM, Miller RM, Strand EA (1995). Management of Speech and Swallowing Disorders in Degenerative Disease. Tucson, AZ: Communication Skill Builders.

Yorkston KM, Strand E, Miller R, Hillel A, Smith K (1993). Speech deterioration in amyotrophic lateral sclerosis: implications for the timing of intervention. Journal of Medical Speech/Language Pathology 1(1): 35–46.

Yorkston KM, Strand EA, Kennedy MRT (1996). Comprehensibility of dysarthric speech: implications for assessment and treatment planning. American Journal of Speech-Language Pathology 5(1): 55–66.

Chapter 7
Changing ideas in apraxia of speech

NICHOLAS MILLER

Introduction

This chapter starts from the premise that past models of acquired motor speech disorders have largely failed us as regards explaining the speech we perceive as apraxic and giving firm indications for differentially diagnosing apraxic speech from other claimed speech disorders. To overcome the impasses and flaws of earlier approaches, a complete revision of our conceptualization of acquired motor speech disorders, and the position of apraxia of speech (AS) within this, has been advocated (Rosenbek and McNeil, 1991; Weismer and Liss, 1991; McNeil, Robin and Schmidt, 1997). This chapter aims to sample some of the debates that exist in this area. There is not room to tackle and give answers to every issue, in as far as any definitive list of issues and answers exists anyway at present. The aim is more modest – to review some main drawbacks to previous ideas about AS; to try to pinpoint key questions that theories of speech production must address to avoid previous impasses; to briefly sketch some of the current directions towards accounts of speech control that might inform debates about AS; and in turn to relate these to our understanding of AS, its assessment and rehabilitation.

Why the need to change ideas on apraxia of speech?

A typical definition of apraxia of speech (AS) prevalent in the 1970s and 1980s spoke of a disorder in programming the positioning of speech musculature and the sequencing of muscle movements for the volitional production of phonemes (Darley, Aronson and Brown, 1975). AS was assumed to contrast in the taxonomy of acquired motor speech disorders with the dysarthrias, considered to reflect neuromuscular dysfunction, and phonemic paraphasia, argued to stem from a phonological deficit.

This perspective grew from models that envisaged separate levels succeeding each other in the genesis of word and speech production. A semantic lexicon fed forwards to a phonological lexicon, which added abstract specifications of sounds and their positions in an utterance. These in turn mapped on to motor commands, providing instructions for muscle movements to produce speech. Breakdowns in the phonological level resulted in phonemic paraphasia, problems with the motor commands produced the phonetic disorder AS and deficits in the transmission of nerve impulses and/or muscle contraction gave dysarthria.

From these levels and associated definitions workers derived lists of characteristics of AS that (should) separate it from the speech features of other disorders. Apraxic speech was said to be characterized by a predominance of perceived sound substitutions (*ben* for *pen*) which differed minimally from the target; phonemic paraphasia was said to show anticipatory, perseveratory, transpositional derailments and substitutions distant from the target (*len* for *pen*; *pay plen* for *play pen*); and dysarthric speech contained mainly imprecise, distorted sounds (Johns and Darley, 1970; Dabul, 1979). Further dissociations were claimed in AS between (relatively) error-free automatic speech and errorful volitional output; speakers were said to evidence struggle in attempts to target a sound or word; error totals increased with longer words and more complex syllables.

However, this view has been demonstrated to be at best incomplete and at worst totally flawed. This has prompted reappraisal of definitions of AS, and its relationship to putative neighbouring disorders dysarthria and phonemic paraphasia. The following sections review some of these (potential) flaws.

Did the claimed features of AS distinguish it from other speech disorders?

The main problem with the features claimed to characterize AS and differentiate it from other aetiologies was that they failed to do so. Perceived speech errors do not reliably distinguish apraxic from other speech types. Apart from maybe a lack of displacement derailments (anticipations, metatheses and so on) in dysarthric speech, all disorder types evidence all perceived error types (distortions, substitutions, omissions and so on) (Square Storer, Darley and Sommers, 1982; Odell et al., 1990; Miller, 1995). Perceptual error profiles can be influenced by artefactual variables such as elicitation stimuli and methods, which material is retained for transcription, broad versus narrow transcription and the influence of the listener's perceptual filter (Buckingham and Yule, 1987; Shriberg and Lof, 1991).

Speakers with dysarthria and phonemic paraphasia may also show length and complexity effects (Johns and Darley, 1970; Strand and McNeil, 1996; Nickels, 1997) – not necessarily for the same reasons, but nevertheless rendering the variables unhelpful for distinguishing or explaining what is unique about apraxic speech. Regarding an automatic-volitional divide, quite apart from defining what counts as volitional and automatic, the picture is also unclear. Both paraphasic and apraxic speakers can show the distinction. Likewise, both apraxic and paraphasic speakers show trial and error struggle behaviour, and some forms of dysarthria present with syllable interruptions and fragments claimed to be unique to AS. Some researchers support qualitative differences in the nature of struggle behaviour between groups (Valdois, Joanette and Nespoulous, 1989); others (Miller, 1992) found apraxic and paraphasic speakers could evidence both types of struggle, even in the run-up to the same word.

A major problem has concerned speaker selection criteria and how far these have biased reliability of findings about neurogenic speech disorders (Miller, 1995; McNeil et al., 1997). Varying definitions of AS and unreliable distinguishing criteria have led to difficulty in deciding whether groups in different studies said to represent apraxic speakers are indeed identical and whether contrasting groups have been separated along equivalent lines. Rosenbek and McNeil (1991) invited us to set aside previous assumptions about dysarthria and AS until more reliable data were available, ideally based on studies of 'pure' cases. Of course, this raises the thorny issue of what criteria constitute the definition for a pure case. Either one has to proceed with definitions that are theory bound and always at risk of circularity of argument ('I believe AS shows X, Y, Z. Here are some speakers with X, Y, Z, they must be apraxic'); or, as others (for example, Weismer and Liss, 1991) have advocated, adopt a data-driven perspective, centred on individual speakers, only starting to speak of separate syndromes if clear dissociated groupings eventually appear from clinical populations.

Problems, though, run deeper than these relatively superficial (but still non-trivial) issues. The reason that many of the hoped-for distinctions in perceptual features failed to be watertight on closer scrutiny leads back to more fundamental difficulties in the models of speech production lying behind the claimed taxonomies of acquired motor speech disorders and alleged differentiating behaviours.

Some problems of linear hierarchical models

Despite several variations in the type of hierarchical information processing model alluded to above, all share certain assumptions. A central programme for each word or sound in the lexicon is selected whenever the particular word needs to be said. This central programme contains all the details the speech production system requires to produce the string. Although there are several, serially ordered levels of processing, essentially all the lower levels do is translate codes from the output of the previous level to unpack the instructions for that level to compute. In other words, these models represent hierarchical, top-down, address-specific, discrete point, translation models (Miller, 1989; Kent, 1997). However, research has delivered findings that weaken or contradict claims for central programmes, hierarchically arranged, with address-specific invariant instructions to constant articulators, a strict demarcation between phonological and motor processes, centred around the phoneme and its features.

Perturbation studies (Gracco and Abbs, 1989; Munhall, Löfqvist and Kelso, 1994) indicate that non-central elements of control have a degree of autonomy in altering behaviour and that articulators do not operate in isolation from each other with their own piece of central command. It is logically and neurophysiologically unlikely that the brain could store all the sound production commands a speaker ever needs.

In opposition to a view of strictly divided levels, many studies have established the presence of motor disruptions in contexts or with speaker groups where none was predicted, and vice versa (McNeil et al., 1990, Vijayan and Gandour, 1995; Kurowski, Blumstein and Mathison, 1998). A ubiquitous finding in 'healthy' as well as 'disordered' speech is that a given word or sound may be achieved on different occasions through quite different articulatory means (Edwards and Miller, 1989; Gentil, 1992; Wood and Hardcastle, this volume). There is the parallel observation that the same acoustic signal may be perceived on different occasions as different sounds, while different acoustic output may be heard as the same sound.

The fate of the phoneme as a unit of control has not fared well either. Arguments for the psychological reality of the phoneme as a perceptual unit might be mustered. However, evidence for its existence as a unit of planning or execution is slim. Objections have been raised to the use of phonological features as putative manipulated variables in control (Walsh, 1974). Their arbitrariness is aptly illustrated by the totally different calculations that are made for feature distances depending on which feature system is used. The differences arise because linguistic features are arbitrary units which, notwithstanding claims to the contrary, do not necessarily have any reality in terms of what is manipulated in action control. There is no logical reason from a motor control point of view why the contrast /p/~/k/ should be counted as a two feature difference, but the contrast /p/~/t/ or /t/~/k/ only one. One can describe dysarthric speech in terms of feature changes, but no one would claim on that basis that neuro-muscular changes bring about a phonological disorder, or vice versa. This kind of argumentation is an instance of the false reasoning that confounds descriptive units and products of movement with units of control.

A further flaw is seen in the view of speech control and its disorders that maintains a strict demarcation between phonological and phonetic domains. Fowler and colleagues (1980) saw as a central question for speech motor control accounts, how do hypothesized abstract mental images that are discrete, context-free and static map on to physical actions which are continuous, context sensitive and dynamic – namely, how do the abstract phonological specifications turn into instructions for muscles, nerve impulses, motor acts and movement? Most workers evasively stated that abstract phonological specifications mapped on to motor commands, without a word about where these motor commands might come from, what form they took, how the mapping takes place, how they might accommodate to the differing contexts in which a sound might occur, and so forth. They ignored the challenge of establishing how, within the constant variability of articulatory behaviour, the vocal tract produces an invariant functional goal.

One problem address-specific models face in solving the mental-physical divide is that they embody a mechanistic attitude to speech perception-production. An invariant central programme dictates messages to subordinate, unthinking levels. Lower levels simply unpackage instructions from the cortical homunculus. Articulators do nothing more than respond to the commands. Such systems reflect a theory of reaction, not action. The vocal tract on which commands operate is viewed as a passive recipient of invariant instructions. Decisively, too, the external (to the speaker) environment is deemed inert, constant, and therefore inconsequential to the speech production-perception process. Research demonstrates that neither assumption is true.

A major problem with central commands concerns the fact that they must act on a constantly changing vocal tract. Articulatory configurations vary, depending on preceding and upcoming sounds. 'Instructions' to muscles also vary for many reasons. On different occasions totally different muscles may be involved in producing a sound, or the same muscles, but in a completely different relationship to each other. Muscles involved alter according to the starting point of an articulator's movement, the speaker's posture (lying, standing and so on), whether there is food or a cigarette in the mouth and so forth. A given excitation to a muscle produces a different outcome according to whether the current status of the muscle is rest, contraction or relaxation. Heavy structures (muscles, bone, tissues) require different forces to move and halt them than lighter ones. Inertial and reactive forces from movements in other muscles affect control too.

Physiologically, there is no one-to-one relationship between a central efferent 'command' and its effect at the periphery. In a moving body the time lag between central message generation and peripheral arrival means that by the time the message reaches the periphery, the state of the periphery will have changed. Efferent commands can only ever be effected via an afferent context. As such, action must always be under mixed motor-sensory control. Separating afferent and efferent processes will always diminish an explanation of action control, since it is this interaction that embodies the nature of relations between postures. As any central command is meaningless without recourse to the context of its genesis and realization, interaction maintains a focal part in understanding action control.

This emphasizes that motor control, and speech production as an example of this, is not effected within a framework of equilibrium within the speaker, nor between the speaker and environment. Far from invariance being the rule, speech production takes place against the backdrop of constant variability. The goal of actions might be constant (for example, saying a given word at an acceptable level of intelligibility), but the path to that goal can be infinitely variable. A perspective that solves the impasses of previous attempts at characterizing the principles and processes of speech production should therefore include accounts for how an invariant goal may be achieved against the ever-changing state of the vocal tract and speaker–listener interaction.

A further drawback seen in address-specific models concerned their reductionist nature. One level or stage of production was seen as arising directly, linearly from a previous one. Prior stages could be described, and, it was maintained, explained in terms of elements of a more fundamental level. By tracing back through the levels one would eventually arrive at the key to the whole system. By analysing the system down to its most basic constituents one would be able to unlock the secret of its workings. The analysis of speech here is grounded in a theory of things, of objects (phonemes, muscles and so on). Speech is seen as depending on the successive movement of various muscles/articulators, driven by specific commands to specific muscles. If one could pinpoint the basic constituents of phonemes or the primary constituents of the central motor commands, one would unlock the secret of control.

However, to believe that the secret of speech lies in some eventual final component from which all other components are built, and can be unlocked by understanding these individual components of production, is akin to believing the secret of flight or driving can be discovered by describing or analysing the mechanical bits of a plane or car down to their smallest atoms. A theory of things will never deliver an explanation of why a plane flies nor how a car drives along the road. The solution lies in a theory of relations.

The secret of flight, driving and speech is not to be found in any one component. Various mechanisms, or movements, play a part in actions, but this does not necessarily mean that they are components of that action, or hold the secret to the control and success of the actions. Movements have no meaning by themselves, they only acquire meaning in the context of how they interact with other movements towards some functional goal. For instance, the role of lip movements in speech only becomes apparent in conjunction with velum and laryngeal movements, determining whether lip closure is perceived as /m/, /b/ or /p/.

Units of things may be described or analysed hierarchically, but understanding variables in relations between units is possible only through an analysis of interlocking whole parts. Flight only emerges as a product of the interaction of all the components together, and, vitally, of the interaction of these components with external conditions. Flight, driving and speech emerge as products of interaction across a complex set of interlocking parts, but a listing of those part will not furnish an explanation, since the product of that interaction is greater than the simple sum of the parts.

This suggests that a direction for explanations of speech production and its breakdown is in a theory that explores relationships and the products of relationships rather than the behaviour of isolated things. The direction required needs to consider not just forces emanating from command processes of the speaker, but also how these forces are shaped and controlled in the context of biomechanical factors impinging on production, the constantly changing state of the organism as actions unfold, and listener and other environmental variables that influence the perception and production of speech.

Functional synergies

None of these problems and challenges is new. Indeed, it is remarkable that such problems should have arisen in the 1970s and 1980s, since precisely the same problems and attempts to resolve them were formulated in the 1930s by the Soviet physiologist Bernstein (1967). He had been trying to arrive at a viable characterization of the control of any action, not just speech. A key factor he saw to be explained was the degrees of freedom problem. How, given the multitude of parts of the body that need to be controlled separately, the myriad postures and movements the body is capable of producing, does a person manage to restrict output to actions appropriate to the goal of the moment?

The solution Bernstein and his co-workers chose was where primacy was given to defining how a varying set of movements could achieve an invariant action goal; where preset programmes gave way to an (inter)active dialogue between afferent and efferent impulses in the ongoing control of innervation to reach the desired functional outcome of an action. Bernstein emphasized the centrality of the functional task to be achieved. Hence, goals of behaviour were central rather than the mechanical description of individual components of a task divorced from their role in achieving an overall goal. He emphasized explanations based on interaction and emergent properties of systems rather than

inferences about the whole from isolated behaviour of a single component. He conceived of actions as functionally specific, but not anatomically, mechanistically constant; and as the outcome of a dynamic
interweaving of movements ever responsive to the changing demands of
the internal and external contexts of their realization, not the result of
concatenating a series of static postures planned independently of the
context of the task. Bernstein arrived at the idea of the functional
synergy, or coordinative structure, as developed in contemporary action
theory and dynamic systems theory (Kelso, Saltzman and Tuller, 1986;
Saltzman and Munhall, 1989).

Coordinative structures are muscle linkages, often spanning several
joints, that are constrained to act as a single functional unit. Thus, for
example, in reaching out for an object, address-specific models suggest
that shoulder, upper- and fore-arm, wrist, hand and fingers are all
controlled separately. In theories developed around coordinative structures they are deemed to be tightly constrained to act in concert with
each other. Rather than the lips operating independently of one another,
or the jaw, tongue and lips being controlled entirely separately, a
functional synergy perspective views them as being constantly tuned and
retuned to each other to effect the desired functional goal.

Coordinative structures are conceived as having certain qualities
which recommend them as solutions to the degrees of freedom and
variability problems. They are said to possess equifinality – that is, from
any starting position, a synergy will always automatically adjust itself
(without any central executive intervention) to the same final resting
point. This is achieved because of the setting inherent to the synergy,
termed its equation of constraint.

Clearly, any action will involve multiple coordinative structures. A
further property of coordinative structure systems is that when two or
more synergies interact, they come to influence each other's behaviour,
such that they perform as one. They are said to become mutually
synchronized, or entrained (Tuller, Fitch and Turvey, 1982). This intro-
duces a degree of predictability into the system, without having to
postulate central executives to control every aspect of movement. For
speech one might envisage coordinative structures centred around the
larynx, lips, velopharyngeal port, and mandible, with speech produced
by functionally appropriate ennestings and entrainment of these synergies.

What, though, are the functional synergies organized around? To say
lips, velum and so forth indicates nothing about how auditory goals
might be achieved or how the settings for synergies might be determined. A candidate perspective on how the posited coordinative structures of the vocal tract might be organized is offered by the quantal
theory of Stevens (1989) and the related ideas of distinctive regions and
modes proposed by Mrayati, Carré and Guérin (1988).

Organizing functional synergies

Quantal theory demonstrates that perceptually acceptable tokens of sounds are not achieved through an invariant spatial target. Differing configurations of the vocal tract can result in the same perceived sound. Thus instead of there being a prescribed, closely determined, fixed positioning of the articulators, and rigid place features for a given sound, there is greater or lesser leeway for variability of the articulatory targets achieved. Constrictions or closures for a given sound can vary within a given window and still be perceived as the target.

However, at some point in the adjustment of the articulators in relation to each other, there arises a crucial (quantal) boundary. Even though there can be appreciable variation in where articulators are set within the quantal boundary and still be heard as a given sound, at quantal boundaries the slightest adjustment in constriction configurations becomes perceived as a different sound. One might conceive of coordinative structures organized around the distinctive regions and modes or windows for a given language. Equations of constraint are set to maintain the quantal boundaries.

So far this says something about how movements might be constrained to reach a goal, but nothing about how movement might be organized. A possible candidate for accounts of speech control compatible with quantal theory and coordinative structures is represented by gestural phonology (Browman and Goldstein, 1992; Saltzman and Munhall, 1989; Löfqvist, 1990; Kröger, Schröder and Opgen-Rhein, 1995). The key difference between gestural phonology and phonologies associated with the address-specific ideas covered above, concerns the quality of the units of description and control. Rather than abstract linguistic feature specifications, the primitives of articulatory phonology are the basic gestures carried out by the speech production apparatus, that is, sequences and combinations of opening and closing or constriction at different points along the vocal tract, and the changes in rate and power of these movements.

The phonological specification of an utterance is described as a gestural score. This score is written on a number of tiers corresponding to articulatory dimensions deemed to be controlled relatively independently of each other – for example, larynx, velum, tongue, lips. Other tiers are hypothesized to include a rhythmic tier concerned with stress patterning through specification of stiffness and constriction settings and an oral projection tier involved in the ennesting and entrainment of closely linked oral movements. Sounds are described in terms of the relative settings (open, constricted, closed) on these tiers, and, crucially, sequences of sounds are defined in terms of the relative onset, duration and offset of the multiple gestures across different tiers. The relationship between opening and closing gestures is specified not in real time, but in terms of the relative phasing of events. Vitally, relative phasing remains constant over changes in rate and loudness of speech. These latter scalar changes are specified in the gestural score through changes to the velocity and amplitude of gestures.

Figure 7.1 provides a schematic representation of part of the gestural score for 'boot', illustrating different tiers and diagrammatically showing the relative states of open-closed of different articulators at different stages in the utterance. If the time-course of the utterance were to be altered, the absolute time given movements take would be shorter or longer, but the onset and offset of gestures would occur in precisely the same place relative to the movement of other articulators – the different articulators are constrained to act in concert with each other.

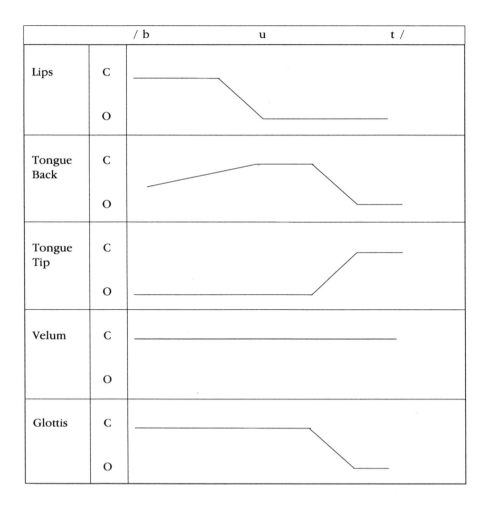

Figure 7.1: Schematic representation of part of the gestural score for 'boot'.

Selecting sounds

There remains still the question of how a speaker knows which sequence of sounds must be produced, and which coordinative structures to select. There are no clear answers to this yet, although within motor control research strong arguments and experimental findings support the view that actions may be directed by perceptual, sensory goals, not motor units (Löfqvist, 1997; Coleman, 1998). What are some of the arguments in this direction?

In action systems articulatory gestures may be set to achieve some temporal-spatial goal within a quantal boundary, but gestures are not constants. Gestures do not define steady states, simply because there are no articulatory constants for a given sound or sound sequence. Instead of being defined in terms of static postures, gestures are inherently dynamic and adaptive. They represent trajectories that unfold in time, and that need to be constantly adjusted along the way. Hence, one argument is that if there are no fixed articulatory goals, then the constants must be the auditory goals a speaker must reach to maintain intelligibility. In speech terms this would indicate a central role for auditory targets in action control, with articulators guided on-line through multiple, integrated efferent–afferent loops, and constant feedforward and feedback.

Another argument used to support the primacy of auditory targets is the elusive search in brain imaging studies for a phonological output lexicon. This remains a contentious area. The core of the argument centres around tasks believed to involve activation of how whole word forms should be said. Motor-based theories of articulation and ideas of an independent phonological lexicon containing programmes for spoken word forms would predict activation coincident with whole words, predictably in (left) frontal motor areas. Currently, the weight of evidence (Coleman, 1998) lies towards there being an auditory-based lexicon, a memory store of the acoustic shape of a word centred in the left superior temporal lobe, but no articulatory lexicon.

These auditory memories are argued to serve as stimuli for assembling coordinative structures to realize target sound strings. But the coordinative structures are most likely not word specific – there is not some separate, specific coordinative structure stored and recalled for every word. Indications are that programming is based on sublexical units. Whether some routines might be stored and recalled as needed while other synergies are constructed anew to serve the specific context, also remains debatable (Keller, 1987). This represents a key contrast with central programme hierarchical models. Rather than fixed central motor programmes for each word, production here is directed towards an auditory target, with movements assembled to fit the prevailing articulatory context, and with construction and execution monitored and controlled on-line through constant efferent–afferent loops that ensure that the unfolding, emergent sound pattern is moving towards the desired acoustic effect.

Another argument mustered to support a single auditory-based phonological lexicon comes from aphasia studies (Coleman, 1998). If there were independent neuroauditory and neuromotor lexicons one might expect to find speakers with aphasia where one but not the other is affected. In particular, if the auditory memories could be impaired independent of an output store, one would predict speakers with impaired (spoken) word comprehension but appropriate word selection and fully intelligible speech. Such cases are not reported. Speakers with pure word deafness seem to fit this description, but it still has to be proven that this is a disorder of word perception and not a more general phonetic impairment affecting non-lexical speech (Allport, 1984). The few studies examining non-lexical phonetic perception (for example, Saffran, Marin and Yeni-Komshian, 1976; Auerbach et al., 1982) seem to indicate that such a disorder does underlie pure word deafness.

Some implications for understanding AS

Controversy continues concerning the above debates and their potential relevance and compatibility with each other and to our understanding of AS. Work is still very much 'in progress'. It is not possible to deliver a definitive interpretation of AS within these frameworks. It remains easier to say what AS probably is not than what it definitely is. Concurring with Weismer and Liss (1991), it seems true that pursuing the search for the secret of AS in reductionist models will yield no answers. Reflecting the views of Müller (1992) and Coleman (1998) it also seems true that models based on arguments that ignore anatomical, neurophysiological reality will not benefit us. Despite the absence of firm conclusions, some tentative hypotheses might nevertheless be ventured and possible reinterpretations of known features of apraxic behaviour be offered.

We can say some things that might underlie AS from the above descriptions, in as far as aspects of production can be identified that could dysfunction. Whether in a completely interactive, integrated system one can ever speak of independent, strictly delineable syndromes or units (for example, ataxic dysarthria vs AS vs phonemic paraphasia; phonemes, features and so on) remains an empirical question. Also problematic in interpreting behaviours in a self-regulating system is the distinction between core and compensatory symptoms.

Core symptoms reflect the direct effects of a damaged/missing process. Compensatory symptoms are manifestations of the way in which output has been (unconsciously, consciously, or both) modified to cope with an underlying deficit. In a self-righting system, the changed behaviour one views when a component is malfunctioning is not the rest of the system working as normal, minus that function. Rather, the changes reflect the working of the system reorganized to function without the particular component – or, as Bernstein (1935:84 in Whiting, 1984) formulated, a movement never responds to detailed changes by a change in its detail; it responds as a whole to changes in each small part. Such changes may be reflected in phases and details distant both spatially and temporally from initial perturbations. Hence, in some respects, all perceived changes might be termed compensatory. Untangling such knots must await further research (Clark and Robin, 1998). Mindful of these unresolved questions, the following paragraphs consider some of the variables, and their disruption, that might underlie what we perceive as apraxic speech.

Within the directions sketched out, a central determinant of what is perceived as disordered speech is the loss of the ability to control the degrees of freedom in the system, the inability to bring the inherent variability in the system under sufficient control to keep movements within quantal target boundaries. The following paragraphs consider how aspects of this loss may lead to perceived distortions, substitutions, omissions, additions and displacements, as well as other behaviours claimed to characterize apraxic speech.

Crucial in the above scenario for producing normal-sounding speech are the appropriate adjustment of coordinative structure settings, correct phasing of movements and the appropriate scaling of movements in terms of velocity and amplitude. Speculatively, if the phasing between gestures is disrupted or there are problems with the accurate specification of scalar variables, then derailments of one kind or another must come about.

One might predict perceived substitutions when phasing is out to a degree where the perceived sound crosses a quantal boundary. Distortions could arise when misphasing pushes sounds close to a quantal boundary, or when scalar aberrations result in atypical length, loudness, aspiration and so on. As regards omissions and additions, gestural phonologists argue that there are no true omissions or additions – perceived omissions or additions of sounds only represent more extreme alterations to the phasing of gestures. Additions arise when gestures become so uncoupled and elements from other gestures intrude so that a new sound is heard; omissions arise when gestures overlap to such an extent that one masks the other.

Additionally, scalar errors may cause under- and overshoot of gestures which become perceived as additions or omissions. Disruption of scalar changes would also produce perceived distortions and substitutions and could account for some other changes heard in apraxic speech – for example, prosodic features dependent on rate and loudness variation. Disrupted scalar changes could also lead to equalization of stress, atypical stress assignment and problems with rate variation.

Gestural phonology actually postulates that many of the functions mentioned, such as rhythmic make-up of an utterance, consonant–vowel overlap, and control of different articulator groups, are written on different tiers of the gestural score. If such tiers have any kind of explanatory adequacy, then they might be used to predict possible dissociable breakdowns in articulation and a revised taxonomy of neurogenic speech disorders.

Loss of the facility to control the necessary degrees of freedom can help explain some further features of apraxic speech. If an impaired production system can only cope with a reduced number of degrees of freedom, then some of the consequences are that, consciously or subconsciously, a speaker uses units that require less complex control.

The reported tendency to simplification of gestures in AS is one candidate. The universally reported difficulty effecting transitions between postures could derive from the same inability to control the multiple changes necessary to achieve smooth progression. One source of effortful trial and error behaviour could be seen as a consequence of the struggle to organize or set coordinative structures and achieve transitions between postures. Insertion of a schwa, a tactic often adopted in therapy or a strategy some speakers discover for themselves, presumably works because this eases the number of degrees of freedom to control in transitions or prolongs transition times, thereby giving the underfunctioning system time to realize targets without impairing intelligibility. Length and complexity effects are interpretable as consequences of a reduced ability to control multiple gestures at any one time or in succession (Strand and McNeil, 1996; Baum, 1998).

Alterations to (some researchers even assert the loss of) coarticulatory cohesion is a frequently mentioned feature of AS (Buckingham, 1998 for overview; Baum, 1998). Coarticulatorily integrated speech demands the efficient control over multiple degrees of freedom. Loss of this control may cause alteration to coarticulation as a core symptom. Compensatory uncoupling of coarticulatory cohesion to facilitate fluent speech production by effecting speech through a reduced number of degrees of freedom would lead to the same perceived effect. Syllabification and loss of normal fundamental frequency declination fit in here, too (Kent and Rosenbek, 1982). A speaker may be obliged by the severity of the core symptoms to proceed on a syllable-by-syllable basis. Alternatively, through syllabification a speaker may be able to compensate by speaking in units of utterance control that they are able to manage.

Typically, one finds that speakers with AS who speak very slowly or rely on two-word utterances and simple syllable structures can under certain circumstances increase rate, manage multisyllable words without syllabification and tendency to equalization of stress and intonation contours, and produce words with complex syllable structure. This can be partly a function of the automaticity of production – in turn assumed to depend on factors such as frequency in the language of the particular sequence of sounds/syllables and frequency of the word. Another source of such variability, though, may be the trade-off between elements of control that can exist where compensatory tactics are possible in a system.

These improvements, though, usually come at a cost. Enhanced performance in one domain (for example, rate) is traded off against accuracy at syllable or segment level; production of complex syllable words may be gained only at the expense of rate or length of utterance (Clark and Robin, 1998). A similar trade-off interpretation has been offered for morpho-syntactic variability in speakers with agrammatism (Tesak, 1994; Bastiaanse and Jonkers, in press).

The (loss of) degrees of freedom control interpretation of apraxic speech and idea of compensatory trade-off offer a possible understanding of the variability-consistency phenomenon (Deal and Darley, 1972) claimed in apraxia. The complexity of a particular sequence of postures and how to achieve the target ennesting and entrainment of synergies remain a constant hurdle for the speaker – hence consistency in where derailments arise. However, because the solution to the problem, the way in which compensation is sought or the way in which the phasing and scaling breaks down are not constant, variability of realization arises, causing listeners to perceive first a distortion, now a substitution, now a deletion even for the same sound (combination).

Where might derailments arise?

Postulating that underlying problems stem from impairment of organization of coordinative structures and loss of control of the degrees of freedom is only a direction for solutions. It still begs the question of how do breakdowns occur. This section briefly considers some candidate concepts for underlying impairment. Firm conclusions await clarification of many of the theoretical issues alluded to and investigatory confirmation of their clinical validity.

In the above scenarios a first step hypothesized would be formulation of the functional goal (or 'model of future need', as Bernstein terms it). Coleman (1998) makes a strong case for this occurring through access and retrieval from memory of the auditory form of a word. The exact nature of these 'memories' remains unclear, but they are likely to be far from traditional separate, abstract, canonical, normalized phonological dictionary entries for each word, with details of the output specifications needed to produce that word. Goldinger (1997), among others, has argued in favour of an episodic, exemplar based auditory memory, where mapping from the speech signal to representation is simple, but representations are complex. This contrasts with views that see abstraction of normalized features from a highly variable signal as complex, but representations as simple. The same may apply to production.

These auditory lexical representations are transformed into articulatory plans, based on recruitment of coordinative structures that again most likely are not based on word units. Browman and Goldstein's articulatory phonological theories provide a possible framework for specifying the implementation of gestures, their ennesting and entrainment, with specification of the phase relationships and scalar values of production. The coordinative structures would be set to target configurations within the quantal boundaries compatible with achieving the target auditory effect. Another vital constituent is the constant afferent–efferent dialogue within the system, both internally and to the external context.

Within this formulation one might predict that underlying impairments could arise from problems in specifying the model of future need, access to, retrieval of and/or integrity of auditory memories and holding these in short-term memory long enough for comparison during translation to articulatory score and execution (Schwartz et al., 1994; Hough and DeMarco, 1996). Retrieval may be impaired by an imbalance in activation-inhibition within the system (see below) and translation and subsequent control may be affected by disruption to the online feedback matching. Lack of awareness of listener feedback also constitutes a potential source of faulty output tuning. If there is a repertoire of stored functional synergies, then conceivably speech production could be impaired by deficits in storage or retrieval. If synergies are constructed de novo, this too would represent another node of possible breakdown. A cluster of impairments may centre around the specification of the gestural score and equations of constraint for the ennesting and entrainment of coordinative structures and realization of the correct relative timing between gestures (Clark and Robin, 1998).

Another issue concerns how utterances are read off perceptually and controlled articulatorily. Within an interactive activationist system (Dell and O'Seaghdha, 1992; Müller, 1992) probability plays a large part in predicting upcoming (perceptual and production) targets. Where information is predictable from a context, it may be processed in a different manner to contexts where further computation is required to understand or produce an utterance. For instance, in the contexts /ˈelɪf.../, or 'He drank a cup of /ˈkə.../ it may not be necessary to process the rest of the word for understanding, and in production the movement planning for /ənt/ and /fɪ/ may be selected and run off automatically since the remaining movements are entirely predictable from the preceding context. It may be that this is one way in which the planning and execution of movements is achieved in a less costly fashion. By contrast, one would expect different processing in contexts where the upcoming sound sequence is not predictable (in as far as there are not clues from the broader knowledge and meaning context).

Evidence points to on-line monitoring being a significant problem for speakers with perceived apraxic and paraphasic speech (Liss, 1998; Marshall et al., 1998). Because these speakers are generally painfully aware of their production errors, it might be assumed that there exists adequate monitoring of output. However, Liss (1998), from analyses of the loci and time course of self-corrections, argues that even for speakers with 'pure' AS there are derailments from failure to monitor production prearticulatorily. In coincidental support of a view that postulates inter-action across phonological and non-phonological components of production, her participants evidenced linguistic sources of errors, despite no indication of aphasia. The speaker described by Marshall et al. was also unable to monitor self-initiated naming adequately (although he could monitor repetition output), despite relatively good comprehension.

Implications for taxonomies of neurogenic speech disorders

As noted earlier, reformulation of our views on speech production must carry the possibility that at the very minimum the basis of how we differentiate speech disorders from each other will change. More likely, our taxonomy of speech disorders would be radically altered, with divisions along entirely new lines. Space precludes a full discussion of this. The following briefly considers one example of the way rethinking could alter our views.

Interactive activation theories state that elements in emerging systems are not selected on an all-or-nothing basis. For instance, in naming a target picture 'book', not only will 'book' be activated as a candidate for production, but also closely related words such as 'magazine', 'library', 'booklet', 'read'. For each of these candidates there would be activation of close-sounding strings – for example, target 'read' may activate /lid/, /nid/, /rip/. Within an efficiently running system inappropriate candidates are rejected because their threshold is not raised sufficiently by boosts from other (internal and external) contextual cues. If the balance is tipped too far in either direction characteristic pictures emerge.

Increased inhibition (raised activation thresholds) results in only elements that have high resting potentials to start with (and so require only a minimal amount of extra activation) or only candidates that receive extra-large boosts from contextual activators achieving full selection. In practice this usually means elements that require little resourcing – that is, high-frequency elements, ones uniquely or highly predictable from the context, or relatively automatized elements of the language.

This offers a potential explanation for the automatic-volitional divide claimed as characteristic of AS. One source of effortful trial and error behaviour may be the struggle to achieve an underactivated target. The fact that in AS syllable structures tend to be the canonical forms of the language and sound production deteriorates in the direction of (motoric) simplification also fits this picture.

A mirror image stems from insufficient inhibition in the system. Here, unwanted elements competing with the target become activated instead of, or alongside, the desired goal. In these instances one would expect frequent paraphasic intrusions, not necessarily close to the target sound, sound blendings of competing target sounds, and combined semantic-phonemic paraphasic derailments. In other words, just the picture claimed in phonological jargon and phonemic paraphasia.

Hypothetically, the perceived fluent, phonotactically accommodated speech produced in this picture arises because the disruption occurs in the selection from auditory memories and associated disruption to the selection and preparation of coordinative structure plans prior to movement onset. The *conduits d'approche* characteristic of this picture contrast with AS struggle in that they would be predicted to flow from attempts to suppress unwanted intrusions and misactivations, as opposed to shortfalls in activation. Another, or alternative, source of articulatory accommodation may come from the automatic adjustment capability of coordinative structures. Separate lexicons for form versus content words need not be invoked to explain apparent dissociations in where pronunciation derailments occur. Differences would arise as a function of word frequency and word neighbour effects that influence activation and inhibition patterns.

The activation–inhibition distinction gives a possible basis for the distinction for what has been labelled in the past apraxic versus paraphasic speech. However, the distinction here is drawn not from a categorical distinction between phonetic and phonological levels of processing. Instead, the perceptual picture arises from points towards either end of a continuum where the centre point represents a normal balance between activation and inhibition and where the extremes represent disinhibition and overinhibition. 'Errors' traditionally defined as phonological or phonetic derive from the one (impaired) underlying control dimension. Derailments might be classed as phonological or phonetic (just as they can be in the transcription of dysarthric speech), but this constitutes a descriptive distinction imposed on the resultant perceived derailment, not an explanatory account of error genesis.

A further attraction of the activation–inhibition continuum comes from evidence suggesting that it is a neurophysiologically real process. Among others, Frith and colleagues (1991) and Jahanshashi and colleagues (1998) (see below) have pointed to a possible mechanism centred around a loop linking the dorsolateral prefrontal cortex with the superior temporal gyrus. The fact that AS and phonemic paraphasia are found in lesions around this loop lends further support. The same loop may form part of the efferent–afferent on-line control system, with stored auditory memories in the superior temporal gyrus region (Coleman, 1998) linked to articulatory assembly processes in the frontal motor and premotor regions.

Lesion sites associated with AS

Reports have linked frontal, parietal, temporal and subcortical (basal ganglia) locations with AS (Deutsch, 1984; Kertesz, 1984; Marquardt and Sussman, 1984). Clearly, the answer is influenced in part by what one considers apraxia to represent and where it fits in speech control models. Disagreement continues on both counts. Dronkers (1996) offered CT and MRI evidence supporting the centrality of the left insular cortex in articulatory control, an area already indicated as important by others (Ojeman and Whitaker, 1978; Tognola and Vignolo, 1980; Miller, 1989; McCarthy et al., 1993). But to assume in turn that speech praxis is located in the left insula would be erroneous.

Current views of motor and speech programming emphasize the distributed, integrative nature of control, and the unity and complementarity of centre and periphery, sensory and motor (Gracco, 1995; Kent, 1997) and activation and inhibition. Functional and neurophysiological evidence points to individual functions being dependent on numerous areas of brain, while simultaneously individual areas of brain may participate in multiple functions. Even at spinal level single axons of pyramidal tract neurones diverge on to several motor neuronal pools, while there can be convergence on to a single motor neurone from wide areas of motor cortex (Georgopoulos, 1991, for review). Speech production requires not just selection of appropriate sound patterns. All the processes mentioned above combine to produce spoken output. Activation–inhibition, translation, phasing, scaling and so forth are all dependent on multiple cortical-cortical, cortical-subcortical circuits, which coalesce ultimately to produce speech.

Important loops seem to involve dorsolateral prefrontal cortex (DLPFC)-superior temporal gyrus. Frith et al. (1991) argue that the superior temporal gyrus regions are the site of stored word representations and that inhibitory modulation of these areas by the left DLPFC forms the basis of intrinsic word generation. Tasks employing random number generation (Jahanshashi et al., 1998) and silent word generation (Friedman et al., 1998) arrived at similar conclusions. The parietal lobe is identified as an area containing multimodal and multiple coordinate representation of space, and the posterior parietal cortex seems to contain important circuitries for shifting attention, stimulus selection and movement planning. As such it provides a key interface between sensory cortex and motor cortex in the frontal lobes and performs cognitive operations in the sensorimotor transformation process (Andersen et al., 1997).

Obviously, supplementary and primary motor cortex is involved. The latter, though, is now seen to play a much more active role than being merely the start of the final common pathway between cortex via the pyramidal tracts to the lower motor neurones. Contrary to past claims that there exists a one-to-one correspondence between primary motor cortex cells and target muscles and that complex movements (for example, reaching, word production) are planned and executed as a concatenated series of separate movements, evidence points to movements being controlled within a joint coordinate framework (Soechting and Flanders, 1990; Gerloff et al., 1998), arguably analogous to coordinative structures. Further, distinct cell populations may be differentially tuned to varying aspects of a movement – for example, direction and amplitude (Georgopoulos, 1991).

Cortical functions are tightly integrated with subcortical processes. Jueptner and Weiller (1998) in a series of experiments illustrated the importance of basal ganglia-cortical loops. They had participants learn finger movements. During new learning the DLPFC caudate nucleus and anterior putamen were activated. In movement selection the premotor cortex and mid-putamen areas became activated. For overlearned movements sensorimotor cortex and posterior putamen seemed central, but when subjects were asked to focus attention on these automatic movements activation shifted back to the DLPFC-striatum circuit. From a series of line drawing and tracing tasks Jueptner and Weiller concluded that the (neo)cerebellum is involved in monitoring and optimizing movements using sensory feedback. Others have highlighted the role of basal ganglia in amplitude control, switching from one motor programme to another and organization of simultaneous and/or sequential motor programmes for executing an action (Ho et al., 1998). The cerebellum is also seen to have a role in timing (Jueptner et al., 1995) and contributions to higher cognitive functions (Daum and Ackermann 1995).

Activation studies as well as lesion studies (Kurowski et al., 1998) also point to a role of the right hemisphere in speech output beyond the already recognized role it plays in prosody (Blonder et al., 1995). Kurowski et al. found subtle phonetic changes in output not attributable to the generalized effects of brain damage.

Returning to claims for the centrality of the left insula, evidence for the integration of multiple cross-brain circuits in speech production suggests the importance of the left insula may reside not in it being the location of a speech programmer, but in its position at the junction of motor and sensory cortices, interhemispheric pathways and cortical-subcortical loops, making it a relay and/or integration area for multiple intra- and interhemispheric processes.

Assessment

This section considers some implications of the above remarks for AS assessment. Generally, assessment tasks based on the above tenets may not differ radically from previous practices. What does maybe differ is the rationale for tasks and the interpretations of results. That is the focus here.

A view of speech production directed towards functional goals, where control is heavily interactive, both within the speaker and between speaker and listener, would suggest that assessment of speech production is incomplete, even misdirected, if movements are studied only in isolated, static contexts, in one environment and to one functional end. Assessment that views speech production divorced from the context in which it is used must be sterile and misguided.

Accordingly, assessment should include tasks that measure a speaker's ability to achieve and maintain intelligibility (note, not necessarily 'perfect' speech) in tasks that alternate between postures, with speech produced in varying rhythms, at varying rates and loudness, in contrasting contexts, and to differing functional ends. Assessment searches for the level of control of degrees of freedom that a speaker attains within individual coordinative structures and across ennested and entrained groupings. Equally important would be techniques tapping ability to indicate target auditory targets and ability to monitor and adjust performance on-line.

As noted previously, the actual tasks for this are probably very similar to existing methods: producing syllables in single, then alternating strings; in simple then more complex rhythms; in short, simple strings, followed by longer more complex ones; at habitual then time varied rate; in relatively automatic then more and more propositional contexts, adding less familiar words and less predictable successions of sounds and words. What receives added importance following the ideas introduced above is the way in which length and complexity are built up to reflect increasing functional synergy complexity, the stepwise increase in transitional and cooarticulatory complexity, and the systematicity with which the scalar changes are manipulated.

Because the exact taxonomy of neurogenic speech disorders that might derive from the above perspective remains unclear, differential diagnostic considerations currently must concentrate on finding ways to tease out the hypothesized points of breakdown in the production of speech. For those utterances where intelligibility is impaired, does the speaker's main problem lie with identifying functional targets, keeping a balance between activation and inhibition (and if not, in what direction does imbalance lie?), assembling articulatory routines, controlling the degrees of freedom in the system, maintaining target phasing relationships between gestures, effecting scalar changes, or monitoring and adjusting movement on-line?

Therapy

This section considers some implications for therapy raised by formulations aired in this chapter. It is not a comprehensive review of treatment methods. These are amply reviewed elsewhere (McNeil et al., 1997; Cannito, Yorkston and Beukelman, 1998; Miller, in preparation).

According to the view forwarded, speech control is directed towards functional goals, recruiting task-specific coordinative structures, guided by auditory targets and adjusted by ongoing monitoring. Interaction pervades the system, not only internally to the speaker, but essentially, too, between speaker and environment. This gives several pointers for the principles of therapy.

Since targets are functionally specific, it suggests that there is nothing like speech and real words for practising speech and real words. It suggests that practising routines with no direct application in speech will be inefficient at improving intelligibility. Thus, time spent on non-verbal drills, in general, adds an extra hurdle to therapy, since the speaker will still be faced with how to translate non-verbal rehearsal into verbal gains. (In fact there remains some controversy around the relationship of verbal and non-verbal control of the articulators – Robin et al., 1997).

Task analysis approaches to motor (re)learning concentrate on breaking down tasks into presumed component parts, gaining proficiency in each part and then reassembling them. For instance, a speaker experiences difficulty producing /p/, so the therapist concentrates on silent opening and closing of the lips, then trains closure plus build-up of intra-oral pressure, after which practice at burst release is reached, before finally adding sound. Or, drills are conducted that are presumed to be equivalent to speech tasks – for example, blowing and sucking to train velum function. Again, there are indications that dismantling behaviour in this fashion and training (part)-tasks unrelated to the overall functional act, practised in isolation in a way not natural for the functional goal, are inferior to more holistic approaches (for example, Shumway-Cook and Woollacott, 1995). Tasks broken down but retaining the functional integrity of the overall action may facilitate learning in severe impairment.

Views ventured in this chapter suggest that the prime target of articulation should be achieving acoustic targets rather than prescribed articulatory placement. As the aim is intelligible speech and not articulatorily mythical invariant precision, then functionally successful sound production, especially in the early stages of therapy for more severe impairment, wins out over fastidious insistence on fixed ways of producing fixed sounds (Miller and Docherty, 1995). Further, speech being a dynamic, interactive behaviour, emphasis should be on movements and transitions between postures, not isolated static positions. As the environment for sounds is one of constant variability, therapy should be geared towards contrastiveness in all dimensions – articulatory placement, acoustic targets, stress, rate, loudness and so forth.

Thus, as soon as possible, treatment should practise sounds in contrast, with each other, in differing rhythmic contexts. Therapies that simply rehearse isolated sounds or syllables in regular rhythmic strings can be criticized on the same terms that Bernstein criticized earlier theories – one is training mimes – movements without meaning – rather than the ability to assemble movements into wholes to reach varying functional goals. Emphasis on wholes also incorporates the idea of practising utterances with assimilation prepackaged (Miller and Docherty, 1995); or, if this is beyond a person's capability, then use of compensatory strategies to break strings up into manageable, but communicatively still functional, portions.

In fact, studies on motor learning support these contentions (Schmidt and Björk 1992). Quicker learning takes place using simple repetitive drills in blocks in contrast to tasks demanding problem solving and incorporating variability and random targets into practice. However, when it comes to transfer of learning to unpractised environments and long-term retention, the latter schedules prove more successful.

The importance of formulating and retaining the 'model of future need' and gaining information on one's progress towards it is also stressed in motor (re)learning, emphasizing the importance of securing the correct target and internal and external feedback. Selection is improved if contexts are set up in which speakers do not fail (Wilson et al., 1994). Feedback is more effective if it is informative (your tongue didn't reach the top of your mouth), but uncluttered (not 'because you failed to contract the intrinsic muscles sufficiently so your tongue tip didn't reach the alveolar ridge before you had enough breath to build up') (Schmidt and Björk, 1992). Feedback that tells speakers the gross detail to focus on for change, but allows them to discover their own way of effecting that change seems more favourable, suggesting that, where instrumental feedback is available, systems delivering a single, transparent, real-time trace to monitor win out over systems that require speakers to track multiple variables or where the signal to attend to is not immediately obvious.

Assessment should have established whether unbalanced activation and inhibition constitute a problem in production. If achieving sufficient activation is a barrier, techniques that boost activation should be implemented – for example, use of high-frequency words and sound strings, high predictability of upcoming sounds/movements from previous ones, maximization of contextual affordances. If decreased inhibition of unwanted targets poses problems, treatments of choice would be, for instance, those where contextual affordances are reduced to a minimum and only gradually expanded, those where target sounds and words have no or few immediate neighbours, and where word and sound selection monitoring is sharpened.

Central to fluent, intelligible speech is control of the multiple degrees of freedom. Therapy should therefore commence with postures and transitions where all but the minimum number of degrees of freedom are frozen out. As control improves, more degrees of freedom are systematically added. To some extent, traditional therapies that start with an isolated sound, then two sounds in a row, then three, and so on, do this. However, through this fractionation they run the risk of adding hurdles in therapy and losing the holistic, integrated nature of sensorimotor control. Instead, one should ideally commence with complete gestures and gradually introduce greater and greater differentiation into them.

The metrical approach developed by Ziegler and Jaeger (1993) fits this perspective. They advocate introducing words from the start in their appropriate metric form – that is, syllable number and structure, and stress pattern are all retained (by implication including appropriate coarticulation), even if the actual segments are not precisely those of the eventual target. From this globally correct form the finer details of the individual segments are systematically differentiated. The choice of protosyllable is not arbitrary. Ideally, the initial sound is in the same class as the final target, the sequence of articulatory gestures is the same, or as close as possible, to the final form – for example, in terms of opening and closing gestures of glottis, velum, tongue, lips; and direction of movement (for example, back of mouth to lips, lips to alveolum).

Figure 7.2 illustrates the general principles with some stages in arriving at the target word 'mop'. The first step (in this part of the possible series) 'mom' uses a gesture preserving the overall open-close-open direction of 'mop', but holds other variations as far as possible constant. In the succeeding stages, oral resonance, plosion and voicelessness are gradually differentiated out from the more primitive gesture.

Melodic intonation therapy (MIT) has been reported to bring some success for speakers with AS (Sparks and Deck, 1996). Apart from permitting access to control via other activation channels, the success of MIT may come from its emphasis on whole gestures; starting with minimal degrees of freedom; using highly practised words, with their basic metric elements preserved; using prolonged speech which facilitates transitional control; and progressing with gradual differentiation of gestures into greater degrees of freedom to return to normal speech patterns. Likewise the suitability of PROMPT (Square Storer and Hayden, 1989) for speakers with AS may lie in its facilitation of whole gestures and transitions with multiple channels of support for forward planning and ongoing movement.

		mom	mob	mop
velum	closed			
	open			
lip/jaw	closed			
	open			
glottis	closed			
	open			

Figure 7.2: Possible steps towards target 'mop' using metric approach principles.

Conclusions

Speech production models applied to acquired motor speech disorders in the 1970s and 80s, still manifest in many books and certainly in clinical practice in the 1990s, failed to enlighten us on the nature of underlying impairments in AS. They made claims about the manner and units of control and predicted distinctions between disorders that answered neither clinicians' queries, nor long-recognized flaws in the classes of models proposed. Hence, for instance, the perennial despair discerning whether a particular speech sample signified AS or phonemic paraphasia, AS or ataxia; and whether a derailment was phonetic or phonological.

It has been argued here that these problems arose not because clinicians were failing to apply their learning correctly, but because the lesson itself was misleading. There is no quibble with the broad definition of speech apraxia as a disturbance in the programming of movements for propositional speech. What has been debated above is our understanding of what is programmed in speech control, how it is controlled, where apraxia might fit into suggested revisions to taxonomies of acquired neurogenic speech disorders and possible significance in altered perspectives for managing apraxic speech.

It is hoped that the ideas presented point in a more fruitful direction, steering thought and practices out of some previous impasses. However, it should be stressed that, while there is strong logical and experimental evidence to support the contentions, debate remains ongoing and the application of claims from gestural phonology, interactive activation theory and other strands of thought to speech disorders is in an embryological state. Although work in this direction has begun (for example, Weismer, Tjaden and Kent, 1995), deeper understanding of many of the issues awaits refinement of the background theories and further confirmation of their applicability to clinical data.

References

Allport A (1984). Speech production and comprehension: one lexicon or two. In Prinz W, Sanders A (eds) Cognition and Motor Processes. Berlin: Springer, pp.209–28.

Andersen R, Snyder L, Bradley D, Xing J (1997). Multimodal representation of space in the posterior parietal cortex and its use in planning movements. Annual Review of Neuroscience 20: 303–30.

Auerbach S, Allard T, Naeser M, Alexander M, Albert M (1982). Pure word deafness. Brain 105: 271–300.

Bastiaanse R, Jonkers R (in press). Verb retrieval in action naming and spontaneous speech in agrammatic and anomic aphasia. Aphasiology.

Baum S (1998). Anticipatory coarticulation in aphasia: effects of utterance complexity. Brain & Language 63: 357–80.

Bernstein N (1935). Problems of the interrelationship of coordination and localisation. Archives of Biological Science 38: reprinted in Whiting H (ed.) (1984) Human Motor Actions. Amsterdam: North Holland.

Bernstein N (1967). The Coordination and Regulation of Movement. London: Pergamon.

Blonder L, Pickering J, Heath R, Smith C, Butler S (1995). Prosodic characteristics of speech pre- and post-right hemisphere stroke. Brain & Language 51: 318–35.

Browman C, Goldstein L (1992). Articulatory phonology: an overview. Phonetica 49: 155–80.

Browman C, Goldstein L (1997). The gestural phonology model. In Hulstijn W, Peters H, van Lieshout P (eds) Speech Production: Motor Control, Brain Research and Fluency Disorders. Amsterdam: Elsevier, pp.57–71.

Buckingham H (1998). Explanation for the concept of apraxia of speech. In Sarno M (ed.) Acquired Aphasia (3rd edition). San Diego, CA: Academic Press, pp.269–307.

Buckingham H, Yule G (1987). Phonemic false evaluation. Clinical Linguistics & Phonetics 1: 113–25.

Cannito M, Yorkston K, Beukelman D (1998). Neuromotor Speech Disorders. Baltimore, MD: Paul Brookes.

Clark H, Robin D (1998). Generalized motor programme and parameterization accuracy in apraxia of speech and conduction aphasia. Aphasiology 12: 699–713.

Coleman J (1998). Cognitive reality and the phonological lexicon. Journal of Neurolinguistics 11: 295–320.

Dabul B (1979). Apraxia Battery for Adults. Tigard, Oregon: CC Publications.

Darley F, Aronson A, Brown J (1975). Motor Speech Disorders. Philadelphia, PA: Saunders.

Daum I, Ackermann H (1997). Neuropsychological abnormalities in cerebellar syndromes: fact or fiction? In Schmahmann J (ed.) The Cerebellum and Cognition. San Diego, CA: Academic Press, pp.455–71.

Deal J, Darley F (1972). The influence of linguistic and situational variables on phonemic accuracy in apraxia of speech. Journal Speech & Hearing Research 15: 639–53.

Dell G, O'Seaghdha P (1992). Stages of lexical access in language production. Cognition 42: 287–314.

Deutsch S (1984). Prediction of site of lesion from speech apraxic error patterns. In Rosenbek J, McNeil M, Aronson A (eds) Apraxia of Speech. San Diego, CA: College Hill, pp.113–34.

Dronkers N (1996). A new brain region for coordinating speech articulation. Nature 384: 159–61.

Edwards S, Miller S (1989). Using EPG to investigate speech errors and motor agility in a dyspraxic patient. Clinical Linguistics & Phonetics 3: 111–26.

Fowler C, Rubin P, Remez R, Turvey M (1980). Implications for speech production of a gestural theory of action. In Butterworth B (ed.) Language Production, vol.1. London: Academic Press, pp.373–420.

Friedman L, Kenny J, Wise A, Wu D, Stuve T, Miller D, Jesberger J, Lewin J (1998). Brian activation during silent word generation evaluated with functional MRI. Brain & Language 64: 231–56.

Frith C, Friston K, Liddle P, Frackowiak R (1991). A PET study of word finding. Neuropsychologia 29: 1137–48.

Gentil M (1992). Variability of motor strategies. Brain & Language 42: 30–7.

Georgopoulos A (1991). Higher order motor control. Annual Review of Neuroscience 14: 361–77.

Gerloff C, Corwell B, Chen R, Hallett M, Cohen L (1998). Role of the human motor cortex in the control of complex and simple finger movement sequences. Brain 121: 1695–709.

Goldinger S (1997). Words and voices. Perception and production in an episodic lexicon. In Johnson K, Mullennix J (eds) Talker Variability in Speech Processing. San Diego, CA: Academic Press, pp.33–66.

Gracco V (1995). Central and peripheral components in the control of speech movements. In Bell-Berti F, Raphael L (eds) Producing Speech: Contemporary Issues. Woodbridge, Mass: AIP Press, pp.417–31.

Gracco V, Abbs J (1989). Sensorimotor characteristics of speech motor sequences. Experimental Brain Research 75: 586–98.

Ho A, Bradshaw J, Cunnington R, Phillips J, Iansek R (1998). Sequence heterogeneity in Parkinsonian speech. Brain & Language 64: 122–45.

Hough M, DeMarco S (1996). Phonemic retrieval in apraxia of speech. In Robin D (ed.) Disorders of Motor Speech. Baltimore, MD: Paul Brookes, pp.341–55.

Jahanshashi M, Profice P, Brown R, Ridding M, Dirnberger G, Rothwell J (1998). Effects of transcranial magneticstimulation over the dorsolateral prefrontal cortex on suppression of habitual counting during random number generation. Brain 121: 1533–44.

Johns D, Darley F (1970). Phonemic variability in apraxia of speech. Journal Speech & Hearing Research 13: 556–83.

Jueptner M, Rintjes M, Weiller C, Faiss J, Timman D, Müller S, Diener H (1995). Localisation of a cerebellar timing process using PET. Neurology 45; 1540–5.

Jueptner M, Weiller C (1998). Review of differences between basal ganglia and cerebellar control of movements as revealed by functional imaging studies. Brain 121: 1437–49.

Keller E (1987). The cortical representation of motor processes of speech. In Keller E, Gopnik M (eds) Motor and Sensory Processes of Language. Hillsdale, New Jersey: LEA, pp.125–62.

Kelso J, Saltzman E, Tuller B (1986). The dynamical perspective on speech production: data and theory. Journal of Phonetics 14: 29–59.

Kent R (1997). Speech motor models and developments in neurophysiological science: new perspectives. In Hulstijn W, Peters H, van Lieshout P (eds) Speech

Production: Motor Control, Brain research and Fluency Disorders. Amsterdam: Elsevier, pp.13–36.

Kent R, Rosenbek J (1982). Prosodic disturbance in neurologic lesion. Brain & Language 15: 259–91.

Kertesz A (1984). Subcortical lesions and verbal apraxia. In Rosenbek J, McNeil M, Aronson A (eds) Apraxia of Speech. San Diego, CA: College Hill, pp.73–90.

Kröger B, Schröder G, Opgen-Rhein C (1995). A gesture based dynamic model describing articulatory movement data. Journal Acoustical Society of America 98: 2984–7.

Kurowski K, Blumstein S, Mathison H (1998). Consonant and vowel production of right hemisphere patients. Brain & Language 63: 276–300.

Liss J (1998). Error revision in the spontaneous of apraxic speakers. Brain & Language 62: 342–60.

Löfqvist A (1990). Speech as audible gestures. In Hardcastle W, Marchal A (eds) Speech Production and Speech Modelling. Amsterdam: Kluwer, pp.289–322.

Löfqvist A (1997). Theories and models of speech production. In Hardcastle W, Laver J (eds) Handbook of Phonetic Sciences. Oxford: Blackwell, pp.405–26.

Marquardt T, Sussman H (1984). The elusive lesion – apraxia of speech link in Broca's aphasia. In Rosenbek J, McNeil M, Aronson A (eds) Apraxia of Speech. San Diego, CA: College Hill, pp.91–112.

Marshall J, Robson J, Pring T, Chiat S (1998). Why does monitoring fail in jargon aphasia? Brain & Language 63: 79–107.

McCarthy G, Blamire A, Rothman D, Gruetter R, Shulman R (1993). Echoplanar magnetic resonance imaging studies of frontal cortex activation during word generation in humans. Proceedings National Academy of Sciences, USA, 90: 4952–6.

McNeil M, Liss J, Tseng C, Kent R (1990). Effects of speech rate on the absolute and relative timing of apraxic and conduction aphasic sentence production. Brain & Language 38: 135–58.

McNeil M, Robin D, Schmidt R (1997). Apraxia of speech: definition, differentiation and treatment. In McNeil M (ed.) Clinical Mangement of Sensorimotor Speech Disorders. New York: Thieme, pp.286–312.

Miller N (1989). Apraxia of Speech. In Code C (ed.) Characteristics of Aphasia. London: Taylor & Francis.

Miller N (1992). Struggle behaviour as a diagnostic factor in acquired speech disorders. Paper presented at the International Aphasia Rehabilitation Congress, September 1992, Zurich.

Miller N (1995). Pronunciation errors in acquired speech disorders. European Journal of Disorders of Communication 30: 346–62.

Miller N (in preparation). Working with Motor Speech Disorders. Bicester: Winslow.

Miller N, Docherty G (1995). Acquired neurogenic speech disorders. In Grundy K (ed.) Linguistics in Clinical Practice (2nd edition). London: Whurr, pp.358–84.

Müller R-A (1992). Modularism, holism, connectionism: old conflicts and new perspectives in aphasiology and neuropsychology. Aphasiology 6: 443–75.

Munhall K, Löfqvist A, Kelso S (1994). Lip-larynx coordination in speech: effects of mechanical perturbation to the lower lip. Journal Acoustical Society of America 95: 3605–16.

Mryati M, Carré R, Guérin B (1988). Distinctive regions and modes. Speech Communication 7: 257–86.

Nickels L (1997). Spoken Word Production and its Breakdown in Aphasia. Hove: Psychology Press.

Odell K, McNeil M, Rosenbek J, Hunter L (1990). Perceptual characteristics of consonant productions by apraxic speakers. Journal of Speech and Hearing Disorders 55: 245–59.

Ojeman G, Whitaker H (1978). Language localisation and variability. Brain & Language 6: 239–60.

Robin D, Solomon N, Moon J, Folkins J (1997). Nonspeech assessment of the speech production mechanism. In McNeil M (ed.) Clinical Mangement of Sensorimotor Speech Disorders. New York: Thieme, pp.49–62.

Rosenbek J, McNeil M (1991). Discussion of classification in motor speech disorders. In Moor C, Yorkston K, Beukelman D (eds) Dysarthria and Apraxia of Speech. Baltimore, MD: Paul Brookes, pp.289–95.

Saffran E, Marin O, Yeni-Komshian G (1976). Analysis of speech perception in word deafness. Brain & Language 3: 209–28.

Saltzman E, Munhall K (1989). Dynamical approach to gestural patterning in speech production. Ecological Psychology 1: 333–82.

Schmidt R, Björk R (1992). New conceptualisations of practice. Psychological Science 3: 207–17.

Schwartz M, Saffran E, Bloch D, Dell G (1994). Disordered speech production in aphasic and normal speakers. Brain and Language 47: 52–88.

Shriberg L, Lof G (1991). Reliability studies in broad and narrow transcription. Clinical Linguistics & Phonetics 5: 225–79.

Shumway-Cook A, Woollacott M (1995). Motor Control. Baltimore, MD: Williams & Wilkins.

Soechting J, Flanders M (1990). Deducing central algorithms of arm movement control from kinematics. In Humphrey D, Freund H (eds) Free to Move: Dissolving Boundaries in Motor Control. Chichester: Wiley, pp.115–31.

Sparks R, Deck J (1996). Melodic intonation therapy. In Chapey R (ed.) Language Intervention Strategies in Adult Aphasia. Baltimore, MD: Williams & Wilkins, pp.368–79.

Square Storer P, Darley F, Sommers R (1982). Analysis of the errors made by pure apractic speakers with different loci of lesions. In Brookshire R (eds) Clinical Aphasiology. Minneapolis, MN: BRK, pp.83–88.

Square Storer P, Hayden D (1989). PROMPT treatment. In Square Storer P (ed.) Aquired Apraxia of Speech in Aphasic Adults. London: Taylor & Francis, pp.190–219.

Stevens K (1989). On the quantal nature of speech. Journal of Phonetics 17: 3–45.

Strand E, McNeil M (1996). Effects of length and linguistic complexity on temporal acoustic measures in apraxia of speech. Journal Speech & Hearing Research 39: 1018–33.

Tesak J (1994). Cognitive load and the processing of grammatical items. Journal of Neurolinguistics 8: 43–8.

Tognola G, Vignolo L (1980) Brain lesions associated with oral apraxia in stroke patients. Neuropsychologia 18: 257–72.

Tuller B, Fitch H, Turvey M (1982). The Bernstein Perspective II. In Kelso S (ed.) Human Motor Behaviour. Hillsdale, New Jersey: LEA, pp.253–270.

Valdois S, Joanette Y, Nespoulous J-L (1989). Intrinsic organisation of sequences of phonemic approximations. Aphasiology 3: 55–73.

Vijayan A, Gandour J (1995). On the notion of a 'subtle phonetic deficit' in fluent/posterior aphasia. Brain & Language 48: 106–19.

Walsh H (1974). On certain practical inadequacies of distinctive feature systems. Journal Speech & Hearing Disorders 39: 32–43.

Weismer G, Liss J (1991). Reductionism is a dead-end in speech research. In Moore C, Yorkston K, Beukelman D (eds) Dysarthria and Apraxia of Speech. Baltimore, MD: Paul Brookes, pp.245–71.

Weismer G, Tjaden K, Kent R (1995). Can articulatory behaviour in motor speech disorders be accounted for by theories of normal speech production? Journal of Phonetics 23: 149–64.

Whiting H (ed.) (1984). Human Motor Actions. Amsterdam: North Holland.

Wilson B, Baddely A, Evans J, Shiel A (1994). Errorless learning in the rehabilitation of memory impaired people. Neuropsychological Rehabilitation 4: 307–26.

Ziegler W, Jaeger M (1993). Aufgabenhierarchien in der Sprechapraxie-Therapie und der 'metrische' Übungsansatz. Neurolinguistik 7: 17–29.

Chapter 8
Instrumentation in the assessment and therapy of motor speech disorders: a survey of techniques and case studies with EPG

SARAH J WOOD and BILL HARDCASTLE

Introduction

The production of speech involves a complex chain of events beginning with the generation of neural signals in specific parts of the cerebral cortex and ending with coordinated movements of the organs of speech themselves (the respiratory, laryngeal and supra-laryngeal structures) to produce an acoustic signal. In assessing and diagnosing a speech disorder the clinician is faced with the problem of how best to represent relevant aspects of this complex speech chain. Traditionally, such a representation is based on a phonetic transcription system such as the International Phonetic Alphabet, often with the addition of special symbols and modifications such as in the Ext IPA system (Duckworth et al., 1990). The phonetic representation is usually used either to describe the sound qualities of a particular speech item or as a basis for further phonological analysis. There are other, more elaborate auditory-based systems designed for specific purposes, such as the multi-layered approach used by Harrington in his representation of the speech of stutterers (Harrington, 1986) and the system developed by Vieregge designed for cleft palate speech (Vieregge 1978, 1987).

Auditory-based phonetic transcription systems such as these are undoubtedly useful for the clinician because they attempt to represent the acoustic output of the complex speech production process, and that is, in essence, what the listener attends to. It is also, when carried out by a skilled transcriber, a relatively quick and uncomplicated process involving no elaborate instrumentation or complex experimental set-up apart from a good quality tape recorder. It is therefore understandably one of the most important tools of trade that the speech and language therapist is likely to use in day-to-day clinical activities, not only to identify a phonetic disorder but as a basis for further linguistic analysis.

However, an over-reliance on auditory-based impressionistic transcriptions for representing disordered speech has its pitfalls. For the assessment of motor speech disorders such a representation is relatively unreliable, is too abstract for many clinical purposes and, because of the conventions inherent in transcription systems, can actually be misleading. It is not surprising that in the literature on neurogenic disorders auditory-based analyses produce equivocal results, particularly in areas such as differential diagnosis of different neurogenic disorder types. For example Canter, Trost and Burns (1985: 217), in their investigation of the speech sound patterns of anterior and posterior aphasia, state that 'phonological analysis emerges as a tool sensitive to many of the differences'. Their study revealed significant differences with regard to distribution of error types between apraxic speakers (who they considered to have Broca's aphasia) and those with phonemic paraphasic speech. Blumstein (1973: 73), however, in another auditory-based phonological analysis comparing the speech of six people with Broca's aphasia, six with Wernicke's aphasia and six with conduction aphasia, concluded that 'phonological analysis of aphasic speech revealed no consistent differences among the 3 aphasic groups studied'.

Ziegler and Hoole (1989) point to a psychological tendency in auditory analysis for the listener to favour 'categorical' errors (for example, phonemic paraphasias) over 'non-categorical' errors (phonetic distortions). Another problem arises when one tries to compare results from different studies that use different levels of auditory-based representations. For example, an error analysis based on a phonemic transcription could produce very different conclusions from one based on an orthographic or narrow phonetic transcription. Some investigations have even questioned the value of a broad phonemic transcription for the representation of disordered speech where phonetic realizations may be far from normal. In fact, Ball suggests (1991: 61) that 'it is not possible to use a phonemic transcription when you do not know the phonology', which is often the case in severely disordered speech.

The unreliability of auditory-based transcriptions is well documented (for example, by Amorosa et al., 1985; Howard, 1998) and is not surprising given the wide variation in the degree of skill of individual transcribers, their fluctuating powers of attention and the relatively abstract nature of the transcription. In many published reports there is little information provided concerning the background of the transcribers or tests of inter- and intra-transcriber reliability. Another problem is the abstract nature of the representation. Essentially, most conventional phonetic or phonemic transcriptions are segmentally based. While there may be some psychological reality of units such as sound segments and phonemes (Laver, 1994), essentially the transcription is attempting to represent a continuously moving and overlapping series of articulatory events as a sequence of discrete symbols arranged in a linear sequence on the page running from left to right. Instrumental studies have shown, however, that clear boundaries between sound segments cannot always be identified (Fujimura and Erickson, 1997). One consequence of the conventions used in transcriptions is that listeners tend to place sounds into discrete categories, which correspond with those of their native language (Ziegler and Hoole, 1989), leading to what Buckingham and Yule (1987) term 'phonemic false evaluation'. Allied to this is the Phonemic Restoration Effect identified by Warren and Obusek (1971) to account for the fact that listeners' knowledge of the target can affect their perception of speech sounds. They presented to their listeners audio recordings where certain speech sounds had been spliced out but where the listeners knew the target. Listeners reported hearing the sound, which Warren and Obusek took as evidence of a top-down influence connected with the lexical and morphological identity of utterances that can affect perception.

Another problem arising from the abstractions of the segmentally based transcription is that listeners are often encouraged into making categorical judgements of the type: is this an alveolar or a velar plosive, where in actual fact different parts of the tongue may be abnormally contacting both articulatory regions simultaneously, resulting in a sound with acoustic and articulatory characteristics of neither. Such 'double articulation' patterns have been recorded in apraxic speakers (see Hardcastle and Edwards, 1992) and are heard variously as phonemic substitutions or alveolar/velar distortions, depending on which gesture (tongue tip for the alveolar or tongue body for the velar) is released first (see further discussion in Hardcastle and Edwards, 1992). An auditory evaluation is not able to resolve such articulatory events and thus may provide misleading information on the characterization of the disorder in question.

Because of these limitations of auditory-based evaluations, instrumental methods have begun to play an increasingly prominent role in the clinical management of clients with neurogenic speech disorders. Instrumental techniques can provide objective quantitative data on a wide range of clinically relevant acoustic, physiological and aerodynamic features and, for many speech and language therapists today, these data are essential to complement the auditory-based impressions for a more precise diagnosis and assessment. Another spin-off benefit of instrumental techniques is that they can often be adapted to provide real-time visual and auditory displays of relevant speech parameters, which can be used as biofeedback devices for modifying abnormal speech patterns. In their recent comprehensive review of instrumental assessment of the speech mechanism, Thompson-Ward and Murdoch (1998: 68, 69) point to three main stages of clinical management in which instrumental techniques can enhance the abilities of the clinician:

- increasing the precision of diagnosis through more valid specification of abnormal functions that require modification;
- the provision of positive identification and documentation of the therapeutic efficiency: short-term assessment and long-term monitoring of the functioning of the speech production apparatus;
- the expansion of options of therapy modalities, including the use of instrumentation in a biofeedback modality (Baken, 1987).

However, although instrumental techniques provide valuable data for the clinician, they are not without their limitations, and certain prerequisites must be met before they are clinically viable. First, they must be non-invasive, involving a minimum of potential danger or discomfort to the client. Many of the older techniques involving X-rays are now deemed to be inappropriate for routine clinical use because of the inherent danger of radiation damage. Similarly, techniques that involve inserting probes into the nasal cavity or inserting miniature electrodes into the body of muscles may not be suitable for some subjects, although there is minimal hazard to health by using such devices. They do, however, involve some degree of discomfort to the subject and are therefore relatively unsuitable for routine clinical use. For such techniques to be used, it is advisable to have a suitably qualified medical person in attendance.

The second main prerequisite is that the instrumental technique should not appreciably interfere with the speech production process. The degree of interference is sometimes difficult to determine and often a balance must be struck between the potential for interference and the need to obtain specific data. Most techniques that record directly movements of the speech organs inside the mouth involve inserting some sort of foreign body either worn on the hard palate (for example, the artificial palate used in electropalatography (EPG)) or attached directly on to the articulator itself (for example, the magnetic coils fastened on to the tongue for electromagnetic (midsagittal) articulography (EM(M)A). It is often up to the clinician to determine in any given case whether the use of the technique will adversely affect the function of the speech organ and if so, some attempt should be made to quantify this detrimental effect and take this into account in interpreting the results of the analysis.

Third, the techniques should provide measures of speech data which are phonetically and clinically relevant. It is important that the technique provides measures that can be related fairly directly to actual physiological or acoustic attributes of speech production. Many measures, such as, for example, some of the perturbation measures of vocal fold function, need to be interpreted in the light of far more normative data than is available. Also, some of the assumptions made about velopharyngeal function on the basis of nasal airflow measures may well be ill-founded if other factors are not taken into account, such as lung volumes, pressure/flow relationships and so on. When assessing the suitability of a particular instrumental technique it is important to take into account such factors.

Finally, for instruments that enter the oral cavity there are a number of practical considerations (see Stone, 1996: 496). They should be unaffected by temperature change, by moisture and by changes in air pressure. As Stone points out (1996: 496), if adhesives are to be used they should be designed to stick to expandable moist surfaces and be removable without tearing the surface tissue. Table 8.1 summarizes the main features of auditory-based transcription versus instrumental analysis (see also discussion in Gerratt et al., 1991).

Table 8.1: Summary of the main features of auditory-based transcription versus instrumental measures for the representation of disordered speech data

Auditory-based transcription	Instrumentation
1. Quick	1. Relatively time-consuming
2. Uncomplicated	2. Often complicated to use
3. Cheap	3. Relatively expensive
4. Entirely non-invasive	4. Often relatively invasive
5. Does not interfere with normal speech	5. May interfere with normal speech
6. Relatively unreliable	6. Objective and reliable data
7. Abstract representation	7. Precise information on articulatory, laryngeal and respiratory activities possible
8. Segmentally based	8. Represents continuous nature of speech events
9. Encourages categorical judgements	9. May be used in a biofeedback modality
10. Attempts to represent what listener hears	

In this chapter we review some of the main techniques that have been developed for clinical and research purposes. This is followed by a more detailed discussion of one particularly useful technique, electropalatography, in the assessment and treatment of adult neurogenic disorders.

Survey of instrumental techniques

The following section summarizes some of the main instrumental techniques used to investigate activities of the various organs of speech (including supragottal articulators such as the tongue, lips, jaw, soft palate, and laryngeal and respiratory structures). The summary is not meant to be exhaustive. It is simply meant to illustrate the range of techniques available. In the tables that follow, references are given to published sources where further information on particular techniques is available. The reader is referred also to a number of recent reference works which survey instrumental techniques used for clinical and research purposes. These include Baken (1987), Lass (1996), Ball and Code (1997), Hardcastle and Laver (1997), Thompson-Ward and Murdoch (1998), Baken and Orlikoff (in press).

For convenience of description the various techniques are grouped under eight main headings: acoustic analysis, aerodynamic measurement, imaging techniques, movement transduction, pressure/force transduction, mechano-acoustic techniques, tongue-palate contact analysis and neurophysiological analysis. Throughout this discussion we will focus on the application of the technique to the assessment, diagnosis and treatment of adult acquired neurogenic disorders, particularly aphasia, apraxia of speech (AOS) and dysarthria.

Acoustic analysis

Acoustic analysis provides indirect information only on activity of individual speech organs, although algorithms for specifying the relationship between acoustic features and movements of specific organs have developed considerably over the past few years.[1] Table 8.2

Table 8.2: Techniques of acoustic analysis

Technique	Typical measures	Target organs	Further reading
Spectrography	Duration (e.g. VOT, stop gap duration, vowel duration, rate) Fundamental frequency Vocal quality (e.g. jitter, shimmer, harmonic to noise ratio) Formant frequencies (particularly rate and extent of formant transitions) Voicing Aspects of noise spectra	All (indirect information only)	Kent and Read (1992) Orlikoff and Baken (1993) Baken and Orlikoff (in press) Farmer (1997)
Oscillography (wave-form analysis)	Periodicity (indicating voicing) Spirantization Duration (e.g. VOT, stop gap duration, rate)		Weismer (1984 a,b)

summarizes the techniques for acoustic analysis and a sample of the various measures that can be made from the acoustic signal.

Prosodic and suprasegmental aspects of speech, such as timing, rhythm, fundamental frequency variations, as well as qualitative changes indicating different phonation types and manners of articulation, can conveniently be investigated by acoustic analysis and have proved to be extremely useful for the clinician working with acquired neurogenic disorders.[2] The major advantage of acoustic analysis techniques is that they are entirely non-invasive and require only a good-quality microphone and suitable analytical equipment. Acoustic analysis in the clinic has been greatly facilitated in recent years by the ready availability of suitable low-cost speech digitizing software linked to the PC (see reviews of such equipment in Read, Buder and Kent, 1990, 1992, and the description of a new microcomputer-based system for assessment and treatment in Ziegler et al., 1998). Software has been developed to provide visual displays of relevant acoustic features (such as intensity, fundamental frequency and so on) in a form suitable to be used for treatment purposes (for example, commercially available systems such as Visipitch, Speech Viewer and so on).

Aerodynamic measurement

Like acoustic analysis, aerodynamic measurement provides only indirect information on actual activities of individual speech organs. Such measurement is, however, extremely useful in assessing respiratory function in clients with neurogenic disorders, and a wide range of different techniques have been developed (these are summarized in Table 8.3). Important measures include volume velocity of air flow from nose and/or mouth and pressure variations at different points within the vocal tract (see Hoodin and Gilbert, 1989). Inferences about supraglottal activity can be made on the basis of studying details of pressure/flow variations. Of particular interest is Warren's pioneering work (Warren and Dubois, 1964) in estimating velopharyngeal port area on the basis of pressure/flow measurements.

Most measurements of oral/nasal flow involve some sort of specially designed face mask, sometimes with a rubber seal resting just below the nose on the upper lip. Such a mask can distort the acoustic signal, although such distortion is minimized by a circumferentially vented mask (for example, Rothenberg, 1973). Recent surveys of clinical application of aerodynamic measures can be found in Zajac and Yates (1997) and Baken and Orlikoff (in press).

Imaging techniques

Imaging techniques provide the most direct visualization of speech organs that are available. The representation ranges from a direct visual image such as that provided by cine/video photography (often using

Table 8.3: Techniques for aerodynamic measurement

Technique	Typical measures	Target organs	Further reading
Pneumotach	Volume velocity of air flow through nose/mouth	Indirectly all articulators and respiratory structures	Rothenberg (1977) Netsell et al. (1991)
Anemometer (using heated thermistor)	Volume velocity of airflow through nose/mouth	Indirectly all articulators and respiratory structures	Ellis et al. (1978)
Spirometer	Lung volumes, e.g. vital capacity, etc.	Respiratory structures (indirectly)	Baken (1987)
Plethysmograph	Total body volume providing indirect measures of lung volumes	Respiratory structures (indirectly)	Baken (1987)
Pressure transduction (pressure catheters, miniature pressure transducers)	Oral/pharyngeal air pressure Subglottal pressure (directly by tracheal puncture or indirectly from oral pressure)	Oral and laryngeal structures (indirectly) Respiratory structures (indirectly)	Warren (1996) Warren and Dubois (1964) Anthony and Hewlett (1984) Koike and Perkins (1968)

fibre-optic technology when the organ in question is not accessible to direct visualization) to less direct imaging techniques such as X-ray, ultrasonics and MRI (magnetic resonance imaging). Table 8.4 summarizes the main imaging techniques that have been used to investigate speech production processes.

X-ray technology has been widely used over the years to investigate movement of speech organs in both normal and pathological speakers (by, for example, Kent and Netsell, 1975). The great advantage of these techniques is that they enable one to investigate movements of articulatory organs such as the tongue, lips, jaw and soft palate in relation to fixed structures such as the hard palate, pharynx and so on. However, a serious disadvantage is the potential damage to soft tissue by harmful radiation. This hazard severely limits the routine use of the technique in the speech therapy clinic.

Many recent developments in imaging technology have been aimed at devising safe alternatives to X-ray. MRI and ultrasonics offer useful alternatives and are now becoming better established in assessment and diagnosis of speech disorders (see review in Stone, 1997). MRI is limited by the subject having to be recorded in the supine position and by the relatively slow scanning rate (at present the fastest rate is a few scans per second, but there is relatively poor resolution at this rate). Ultrasound

Table 8.4: Imaging techniques

Technique	Typical measures	Target speech organs	Further reading
Cine/video photography	Dimensions of lip protrusion/ rounding Jaw raising/lowering Shape and type of glottal aperture (using high-speed photography	Lips, mandible, vocal folds	Baken (1987)
Fibre-optic endoscopy	Shape and type of glottal aperture Velopharyngeal opening	Vocal folds, nasopharynx	Baken (1987)
Video kymography	Line-scanning of vocal fold vibration	Vocal folds	Schutte et al. (1997)
X-ray – lateral projection (cineradiography, video fluorograpy)	Articulatory kinematics (displacement and timing of all articulations in relation to fixed structures) Laryngeal dimensions Angle between jaws	All laryngeal and supraglottal structures	Ball (1984) Ball and Gröne (1997)
– Xeroradiography	Steady-state postures of all articulators and laryngeal structures	All laryngeal and supraglottal structures	Dicenta and Oliveras (1976)
Magnetic Resonance Imaging (MRI)	Vocal tract anatomy (based on relative tissue density) Tongue posture Velopharyngeal area (mainly steady-state measures)	All laryngeal and supraglottal structures	Westbrook and Kaut (1993) Baer et al. (1991) Moore (1992)
Ultrasonics	Tongue outline in sagittal and coronal planes Tongue kinematics Pharyngeal width	Tongue, pharynx, vocal folds	Stone (1997) Keller and Ostry (1983)

has a fast scanning rate, is safe and non-invasive and offers great promise for examining the shape of the tongue and pharynx in both the sagittal and coronal planes (Stone, 1991). It has been successfully used in the investigation of dysarthric speech by, among others, Keller and Ostry (1983). The ultrasound image, however, is sometimes difficult to interpret and does not usually indicate the outline of the tongue in relation to other fixed structures such as the hard palate.

A number of specialist imaging techniques have been developed for investigating vocal fold function during speech. Fibre-optic endoscopy can be used to view directly both the soft palate and the vocal folds. The vocal folds can be viewed during normal speech by passing the fibre-optic tube through the nasal cavity and positioning it just above the laryngeal vestibule. It is an optical system only and it is normally not possible to quantify the degree of opening of the velopharyngeal port or degree of abduction of the vocal folds. Skill is needed in positioning the tube to obtain the best image and some clients may find the insertion of the device into the nose somewhat uncomfortable.

Movement transduction

The investigation of kinematics in both normal and pathological speech has used a wide variety of different movement transduction systems. These are summarized in Table 8.5.

Most of the techniques involve attaching some sort of sensing device to the articulatory organ under investigation and tracking the sensor during speech production. Generally speaking, tongue tracking instruments tend to be relatively invasive and require either attaching devices directly to the tongue surface (EM(M)A, X-ray microbeam) or the subject wearing some form of artificial palate (glossometry, optopalatography). Less invasive techniques using optoelectronic technology or strain gauges are used to measure movements of the more accessible organs such as the lips, jaw and respiratory structures (for example, ribcage). Monitoring soft palate movement offers particular problems to the experimenter, and the specialized techniques developed to study velopharyngeal function (Nasograph, Velograph, Velotrace and so on) are limited by the discomfort to the subject of having devices passed directly into the nasal cavity.

Vocal fold function is also difficult to investigate directly, but very useful indirect information can be obtained with electrolaryngography.[3] The Laryngograph is safe and convenient to use and has proved to be a valuable tool in the investigation of laryngeal function in adults with neurogenic disorders.

The study of articulatory kinematics (displacement, velocity and acceleration of supraglottal speech organs) is particularly important for the assessment and diagnosis of clients with so-called motor speech disorders such as apraxia and dysarthria (see, for example, Forrest et al., 1991; Ackermann et al., 1993). Optoelectronic systems that track sensors attached to accessible articulators such as the lips and jaw are non-invasive and convenient to use. Such systems can also be used to

Table 8.5: Techniques for movement transduction

Technique	Typical measures	Target speech organs	Further reading
Electromagnetic transduction (Magnetometry)	Anterior–posterior diameter changes (respiratory system)	Ribcage and abdomen	Hixon et al. (1983)
– Electromagnetic midsagittal articulography (EM(M)A)	x–y midsagittal displacements of coils attached to speech organs Velocity and acceleration of organs	Lips, jaw, tongue (soft palate)	Perkell et al. (1992) Hoole et al. (1993) Schönle et al. (1987) Tuller et al. (1990)
X-ray microbeam	x-y displacement of lead pellets attached to articulators Velocity and acceleration of articulators	Lips, jaw, tongue (soft palate)	Kiritani (1986) Westbury (1994) Itoh et al. (1980)
Opto-electronic systems			
– 'Selspot', 'Optotrak'	Movement in 3D space of points attached to speech organs	Lips, jaw	Vatikiotis-Bateson and Ostry (1995)
– Photo-electric glottograph	Area of glottal opening	Vocal folds	Coleman (1983)
– Nasograph	Area of velopharyngeal port	Velopharynx	Dalston (1982) Ohala (1971)
– Velograph	Degree of soft palate elevation	Velum	Künzel (1977)
– Glossometry	Proximity of tongue to photosensors on artificial palate Velocity and acceleration of tongue movement	Tongue	Dagenais and Critz–Crosby (1992)
– Optopalatography (prototype only)	Proximity of tongue to fibre-optic points on artificial palate Velocity and acceleration of tongue movement	Tongue	Wrench et al. (1996)

(contd)

Table 8.5: (contd)

Technique	Typical measures	Target speech organs	Further reading
Strain-gauge and mechanical transduction – jaw and lip transduction	Force generating control capabilities of lips, jaw Movement of lips/jaw	Jaw, lips	Barlow et al. (1983) Müller and Abbs (1979) Baken (1987)
– mercury strain gauge (Whitney gauge)	Circumferential change in ribcage and abdomen	Ribcage, abdomen	Cavallo and Baken (1985)
– strain gauge pneumograph	Circumferential change in ribcage/ abdomen	Ribcage, abdomen	Murdoch et al. (1989)
– 'Velotrace'	Movement of velum	Velum	Horiguchi and Bell-Berti (1987)
Inductance systems (e.g. 'Respitrace')	Movement of chest wall	Ribcage	Sperry and Klich (1992)
Impedance systems – Electro-laryngography ('Laryngograph')	Details of vocal fold vibration (from Lx trace) Fundamental frequency Glottal wave pertubation	Vocal folds	Abberton and Fourcin (1997)

examine velopharyngeal opening, but this involves inserting a probe into the nasal cavity. A variety of systems using strain gauge technology have been developed once again to measure the dynamics of relatively accessible structures such as the lips, jaw, ribcage and abdomen. They usually involve attaching some device to the structure in question and, for the lip and jaw measurement, a specially designed helmet is sometimes worn. More problematic is tracking the tongue because of its relative inaccessibility. EM(M)A and X-ray microbeam are very effective systems for tracking structures, including the tongue in the midsagittal plane, and have been used for the investigation of motor speech disorders (for example, Hirose et al., 1978, 1981; Itoh, Sasanuma and Ushijima, 1979 and Itoh and Sasanuma, 1984 for the X-ray microbeam; Schönle et al., 1987; Katz et al., 1990 and Hoole et al., 1993 for EM(M)A), avoiding the health hazards posed by conventional cine and video X-ray systems. However, the X-ray microbeam is a highly specialized and expensive system, available at present in only one centre (the University of Wisconsin). EM(M)A offers considerable promise but requires the client to wear a special helmet and involves attaching the magnetic coils directly on to the tongue. For certain clients, this experimental procedure may present problems.

Pressure and force transduction

A number of devices have been developed to measure the force exerted by the tongue and lips (see summary in Table 8.6). These systems are non-invasive, easy to use and provide useful diagnostic information on the force-generating capabilities of clients with neurogenic disorders.[4]

Table 8.6: Techniques for measuring pressure and force

Technique	Typical measures	Target organs	Further reading
Iowa oral performance instrument (IOPI)	Tongue / lip force and endurance	Tongue, lips	Robin et al. (1992)
Miniature force/ pressure transducer	Inter-labial contact pressure Tongue force	Lips, tongue	Hinton and Luschei (1992) Dworkin and Aronson (1986)

Table 8.7: Mechano-acoustic techniques

Technique	Typical measures	Target organs	Further reading
Accelerometry	Vibration patterns on tissues	Vocal folds (indirect information on vibration) Nose (indirect information on nasality)	Horii (1983) Stevens et al. (1975)
Nasometry	Nasal / oral acoustic coupling	Nose (indirect indication of nasality)	Fletcher (1970)

Mechano-acoustic techniques

Indirect information of the function of various vocal tract structures can be obtained from mechano-acoustic devices such as accelerometers (see Table 8.7). These are transducers sensitive to variation and can detect resonance in the nasal cavity (indirectly related to perceptual nasality) and vocal fold vibration (by placing the accelerometer on the neck near the Adam's apple). Two accelerometers can be used to calculate a nasal/voice amplitude ratio as an index of nasal coupling (Horii, 1983). The ratio has been employed in a study of disorders of nasality in clients with dysarthria following a cerebrovascular accident by Thompson and Murdoch (1995), who correlated perceptual judgements of hypo- and hyper-nasality with measures from a nasal accelerometer. Other techniques such as nasometry provide indirect measures of nasality, such as 'nasalance' (ratio of oral to nasal acoustic energy), and employ a mechanical separator to record separately energy from microphones placed in front of the nose and mouth during speech (for example, Fletcher, 1970; Karling et al., 1985).

Tongue-palate contact analysis

The main technique used for measuring tongue-palate contact patterns is electropalatography (EPG) (Table 8.8). It is relatively non-invasive but does require the subject to wear an artificial palate. It offers great promise for the assessment, diagnosis and, to some extent, treatment of motor speech disorders and is described at greater length in the final part of this chapter. According to Stone (1996), in her survey of instrumentation for the study of speech physiology, EPG has been 'an instrument of choice when available because it is only minimally invasive yet provides unique information' (1996: 510).

Neurophysiological techniques

Electromyography (EMG) is the main technique for examining details of the electrical potentials associated with muscle contraction accompanying movements of the speech organs (see Table 8.9). Most speech organs have been investigated with EMG techniques over the years (see reviews in Basmajian and De Luca, 1985; Gentil and Moore, 1997) using

Table 8.8: Techniques for measuring tongue-palate contact

Technique	Typical measures	Target organs	Further reading
Palatography – Electropalatography – Palatometry	Distribution and timing of tongue contacts on artificial palate	Tongue (indirect data on tongue movement)	Hardcastle et al. (1991) Hardcastle and Gibbon (1997)

Table 8.9: Neurophysiological measurement technique

Technique	Typical measures	Target organs	Further reading
Electromyography (EMG)	Electrical potentials associated with muscular contraction (amplitude, timing, frequency)	All	Basmajian and De Luca (1985) Gentil and Moore (1997) Rubow (1984)

both surface and hooked-wire electrodes. Surface electrodes are less invasive than hooked-wire ones and are useful for recording electrical activity in those muscles which are situated close to the surface of the skin and are relatively easily differentiated from other surrounding muscles. Unfortunately, this applies to relatively few muscles involved in speech production, so the use of surface electrodes is rather limited.[5]

EMG has been used as a biofeedback technique in the rehabilitation of dysarthric speakers (for example, Netsell and Cleeland, 1973; Huffman, 1978; Rubow et al., 1984). Muscle tension in these clients is monitored directly by surface electrodes placed on appropriate articulatory organs such as the lips, and feedback on muscle tension is provided by audio, visual or tactile modalities (Basmajian, 1979). By self-monitoring muscle tension, patients with abnormally low levels of muscular tonicity can increase tone and so improve speech performance in, say, the production of bilabial stops. In the Netsell and Cleeland (1973) work, a Parkinsonian patient was trained to decrease excessive activity in the levator labial superior muscle by using an EMG biofeedback system with an audio signal as the control modality. In the study by Rubow et al. (1984) a reduction in hemifacial spasm and dysarthria was achieved by providing auditory feedback of frontalis EMG.

In the brief survey above a wide range of different instrumental techniques are summarized and some indication given as to their suitability as clinical tools. EPG has emerged as the technique of choice for many clinicians in the assessment and treatment of a range of disorders where abnormal tongue movement is indicated. To illustrate its application in assessment and therapy of acquired neurogenic speech disorders we will discuss some recent results of studies exploring the use of EPG in this client group.

Case studies with electropalatography (EPG)

As mentioned above, EPG has been used in both the assessment and treatment of acquired neurogenic speech disorders. Originally designed for phonetic research, the technique is now identified as a useful clinical tool recording the timing and location of tongue-palate contact patterns during continuous speech. Analysis of these contact patterns provides insight into possible causes of the speech disorder. For example, it has been suggested that temporal and serial ordering errors are a result of higher-level motor programming deficits, but spatial errors may be due to lower-level motor abnormalities. Such interpretations can aid diagnosis and are important for appropriate therapeutic intervention.

Most EPG studies of acquired neurogenic disorders have focused on the assessment of patients diagnosed with either apraxia of speech (AOS), dysarthria or both (Washino et al., 1981; Sugishita et al., 1987; Edwards and Miller, 1989; Morgan Barry, 1989, 1995; Hardcastle and Edwards, 1992; Goldstein et al., 1994; Howard and Varley, 1996;

Southwood et al., 1997; Howard, 1998). In a recent study, however, Wood (1997) also investigated speech sound errors in acquired aphasia with presumed linguistic origins. Her subjects were variously diagnosed by traditional classification as Broca's aphasic, with or without AOS, conduction aphasic and anomic.

Although EPG studies of acquired neurogenic speech disorders have involved relatively few subjects, many of the findings have been replicated. Table 8.10 summarizes the abnormalities that have been detected through analysis of EPG data.

Table 8.10: Summary of EPG findings from studies of acquired neurogenic disorders

Summary of EPG findings	Disorder type	Study
Increase in the duration of	AOS	Washino et al. (1981)
lingual palatal contacts	AOS	Hardcastle (1987)
	AOS & aphasia	Wood (1997)
	AOS	Howard (1998)
Increased variability of	AOS	Washino et al. (1981)
target gestures	AOS	Hardcastle and Edwards (1992)
	AOS & aphasia	Wood (1997)
	AOS	Southwood et al. (1997)
		Howard (1998)
Increase in the area of lingual	AOS	Washino et al. (1981)
palatal contacts	AOS	Howard (1998)
Identification of misdirected	AOS	Washino et al. (1981)
articulatory gestures not	AOS	Sugishita et al. (1987)
perceived through auditory	AOS	Edwards and Miller (1989)
analysis	AOS	Ingram and Hardcastle (1990)
	AOS	Hardcastle and Edwards (1992)
	AOS & aphasia	Wood (1997)
	AOS	Howard (1998)
Errors in sequencing and	AOS	Washino et al. (1981)
selection	AOS	Hardcastle et al. (1985)
	AOS & aphasia	Wood (1997)
Distortions in target	Dysarthria	Hardcastle et al. (1985)
configurations (reduction	AOS & aphasia	Wood (1997)
and overshoot of target goals)	AOS	Southwood et al. (1997)
Errors not restricted to a single	Dysarthria & AOS	Hardcastle et al. (1985)
manner or place of production	AOS	Hardcastle (1987)
	AOS	Edwards and Miller (1989)
	AOS	Hardcastle and Edwards (1992)
	AOS & aphasia	Wood (1997)
Disturbed temporal overlap	AOS	Edwards and Miller (1989)
in stop-stop sequences	AOS	Ingram and Hardcastle (1990)
	AOS	Hardcastle and Edwards (1992)
	AOS & aphasia	Wood (1997)
	AOS	Southwood et al. (1997)
Syllable segregation in both	AOS	Howard (1998)
speech and non-speech		
movements, suggesting that		
each gesture is made in isolation		

Duration of lingual palatal contacts

One of the earliest published EPG studies into acquired neurogenic disorders was by Washino et al. (1981). They presented an individual case report of a patient with pure AOS, comparing data from this subject with data from a single control speaker. They focused on the patient's ability to articulate the syllable /ta/ in word initial, medial and final positions and in the nonsense sequence /pataka/. Washino et al. (1981) identified both spatial and temporal abnormalities in the neurogenically disordered speech, specifically that lingual palatal contacts were typically made over a longer duration and there was a greater area of contact.

Other researchers have since replicated these results. In his study of a patient with apraxia of speech, Hardcastle (1987) also noted difficulties of temporal integration, which he compared to the speech of stutterers. Wood (1997) found that aphasics in general (and not just those diagnosed with AOS) produced longer alveolar and velar stop closures. Duration of the /d/ closure in 'deer' and the /k/ closure in 'kitkat' over 10 repetitions was measured from the EPG pattern. The aphasic speakers demonstrated increased duration of closure phases when compared with the control speakers.

Similarly, Howard (1998), in her case study of a patient with severe acquired apraxia of speech, noted significantly greater durations compared with two normal speakers. Target utterances were of the form /əCV(C)/. Increased durations were noted for both the entire utterance and also for smaller units, for example individual syllables. Such increases in duration have also been noted in other instrumental studies. For example, Skenes (1987) measured the duration of phrase, target word, initial vowel, medial consonant and second vowel of the target word for nine apraxic and five normal speakers for two stress conditions and two rates of speech. Using wide-band spectrograms she found that the absolute segment durations were longer for apraxic than for normal speakers. Seddoh and colleagues (1996) looked specifically at speech timing in apraxia of speech and conduction aphasia and compared this with normal control speakers. The temporal measures used were stop gap duration, VOT, second formant transition duration for a vowel, steady state vowel duration, and consonant vowel duration. Abnormal temporal control was identified in the speech of both the apraxics and conduction aphasics.

Increased variability of target gestures

Several researchers have noted an increase in the variability, both spatial and temporal, of target gestures produced by patients with acquired neurogenic speech disorders. Washino et al. (1981), reporting on a single patient with acquired AOS, noted that, while the basic pattern for an alveolar plosive seemed to be maintained, the contact patterns seemed to be more variable. Hardcastle and Edwards (1992) noted that all four of their subjects with AOS produced an abnormal amount of spatial variability, and three of the four speakers were considered temporally more variable. Southwood et al. (1997), in their perceptual, acoustic and electropalatographic study of one apraxic speaker, identified EPG patterns that were more variable compared with a normal speaker. Wood (1997) noted an increase in both temporal and spatial variability. This was statistically significant for four of the aphasics (one Broca's with AOS, one Broca's without AOS, two anomics) during closure phase of the /d/ in 'deer', and three subjects (one Broca's with AOS, one Broca's without AOS and one anomic) during the closure phase of the initial /k/ in 'kitkat'. Spatial variability was calculated using the Variability Index (VI) (Farnetani and Provaglio, 1991). The VI allows comparison of lingual palatal contacts over successive repetitions. A single frame, which identifies a fixed point in the speech signal, is chosen. For the alveolar closure in 'deer' this was chosen as the frame of maximum contact, and for the velar closure in 'kitkat' it was the first frame of velar closure. The mean VI value calculated for the aphasic speakers was greater than that for the control group for both the alveolar and velar closures. However, this was only statistically significant for the velar stop in the word 'kitkat'. Figure 8.1 displays this variability during production of the velar plosive. It shows a prototypical frame representing the start of velar closure for the aphasic speakers. The prototypical frame is a summary of the contacts sampled during 10 successive repetitions. Each square represents a single electrode, and the shading (taken from the electrode variability calculation) indicates the number of times an electrode was contacted over 10 repetitions as a percentage. Figure 8.2 is the same prototypical frame produced by the control speakers.

Area of lingual palatal contacts

An increase in the number of lingual palatal contacts made by patients with acquired neurogenic speech disorders has also been noted (Washino et al., 1981; Howard, 1998). Howard (1998), in her assessment of a patient with severe acquired apraxia, noted broader patterns of closure than would be expected for a normal speaker for targets transcribed as having more posterior closure locations.

Identification of misdirected articulatory gestures (MAGs) not perceived through auditory analysis

In their description of apraxic-based speech errors, Hardcastle and Edwards (1992) identified six different error types produced consistently by four apraxic speakers. One of these errors they labelled 'misdirected articulatory gestures' (1992: 296). These were defined as gestures

FM (Broca's with AOS)

	0	0	0	0	0	0	
0	0	0	0	0	0	0	0
0	0	0	0	0	0	0	0
8	0	0	0	0	0	0	0
10	0	0	0	0	0	0	9
10	10	0	0	0	0	2	10
10	10	10	0	0	10	10	10
10	10	10	10	10	10	10	0

MU (Broca's with AOS)

	0	0	0	0	0	0	
2	2	0	0	0	1	2	2
5	2	1	1	2	2	2	4
8	4	1	0	2	3	5	5
10		0	0	0	3		10
10	10	10	0	0		10	10
10	10		0	0		10	10
10	10	10	10	10	10	10	10

CR (Broca's without AOS)

	0	0	0	0	0	0	
0	0	0	0	0	0	0	0
0	0	0	0	0	0	0	0
0	0	0	0	0	0	0	0
1	0	0	0	0	0	0	1
5	1	0	0	0	0	1	10
10	5	0	0	0	0	5	9
10	10	10	9	4	10	10	10

JM (Broca's without AOS)

	0	0	0	0	0	0	
0	0	0	0	0	0	0	0
0	0	0	0	0	0	0	0
0	0	0	0	0	0	0	0
0	0	0	0	0	0	0	5
0	0	0	0	0	0	0	10
10	0	0	0	0	0	0	10
10	10	10	10	10	10	10	10

IE (conduction)

	2	2	2	6	2	1	
6	7	7	7	7	7	4	2
8	8	4	4	2	5		8
8	4	2	0	0	0	3	7
5	0	0	0	0	0	0	5
3	0	0	0	0	0	0	
9	4	0	0	0	0	4	9
10	4	3	3	3	4	8	9

PW (conduction)

	0	0	0	0	0	0	
0	0	0	0	0	0	0	0
0	0	0	0	0	0	0	0
2	0	0	0	0	0	0	0
10	3	0	0	0	0	0	0
10	10	5	0	0	0	5	9
10	10	9	0	0	5	10	10
10	10	10	10	10	10	10	10

FC (anomic)

	0	0	0	0	0	0	
0	0	0	0	0	0	0	0
0	0	0	0	0	0	0	0
4	0	0	0	0	0	0	0
9	0	0	0	0	0	0	0
10	10	0	0	0	0	0	9
10	10	9	0	0	10	10	10
7	10	10	10	10	10	10	10

HJ (anomic)

	1	1	0	0	0	2	
8	2	1	0	0	0	2	
10	4	1	0	0	0	2	10
10		1	0	0	0		10
10	10	1	0	0	1	10	10
10	10		0	0	8	10	10
10	10	10	3	5	10	10	10
10	10	10	10	10	10	10	10

HL (anomic)

	1	0	0	0	0	0	
1	1	1	0	0	0	0	0
5	1	1	0	0	0	1	1
10	1	0	0	0	0	2	10
10	2	0	0	0	0	8	10
10		0	0	0	0	10	10
10	10	0	0	0	10	10	10
10	10	10	10	10	10	10	10

Scale:

	0%
	1 to 25%
	26 to 50%
	51 to 75%
	76 to 100%

Figure 8.1: Prototypical frame indicating the start of velar closure for 10 repetitions (aphasic speakers)

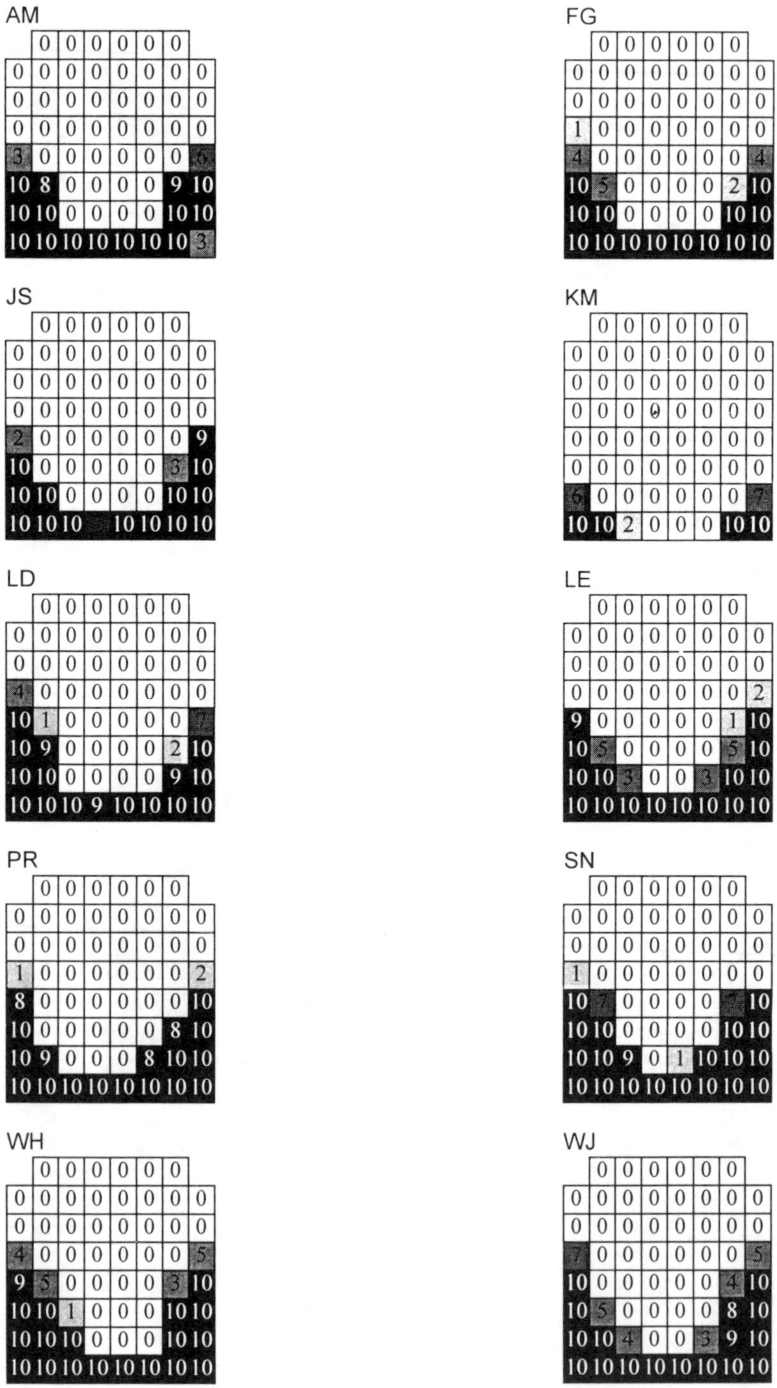

Figure 8.2: Prototypical frame indicating the start of velar closure for 10 repetitions (control speakers)

that were spatially normal but that occurred in an inappropriate place in the target utterance. The most frequent pattern was an alveolar/velar double articulation, which usually appeared in word initial position. Hardcastle, Morgan Barry and Clark (1985) had previously noted these in the speech of an apraxic subject. Typically, the misdirected gesture occurred during production of a word initial alveolar stop closure, for example the initial /d/ in 'deer', 'dolls' and 'dart'. An example of a velar MAG produced by an apraxic speaker (BT) from an earlier study by Hardcastle (1985) can be seen in Figure 8.3. The target gesture /d/ is preceded by full velar closure commencing at frame 0598. Full alveolar closure starts at frame 0606, overlapping with the velar articulation. Therefore, a period of double velar/alveolar articulation results. In this example the velar MAG was variously detected through auditory analysis as [gdɪə] or [dɪə]. These double articulations were also observed, albeit less often, during word initial fricatives ('zoo', 'sheep'). Hardcastle and Edwards noted that the double articulations in 'deer', 'dolls' and 'dart' were 'most frequently ... identified as a normal alveolar stop' (1992: 323) through phonetic transcription and therefore the misdirected velar gesture was unheard. However, if the velar gesture was released after the alveolar this was generally heard.

Sugishita et al. (1987) also identified misdirected gestures that were not detected through auditory analysis in their investigation of omission errors in one left-handed and one right-handed apraxic speaker. On analysis of the EPG data they identified lingual-palatal contacts during perceived omissions. Sometimes the correct articulation had been made but not heard, on other occasions incorrect lingual palatal contacts were detected through auditory analysis. These were similar to those identified by Hardcastle and Edwards (1992) and classified as MAGs since the contact patterns were spatially normal. But unlike Hardcastle and Edwards, who detected intrusive velar gestures, Sugishita et al. (1987) identified alveolar stop patterns.

Both alveolar and velar MAGs were identified in the speech of aphasic adults with and without AOS (Wood, 1997). In her study of 10 neurogenically impaired adults with speech sound errors (two Broca's with AOS; three Broca's without AOS; two conduction aphasics and three anomic aphasics), eight subjects produced MAGs (one Broca's without AOS and one anomic did not). In addition to noting alveolar and velar MAGs, Wood (1997) identified another category, double articulation MAGs. These were defined as articulations where neither an alveolar nor a velar phoneme were the target gesture but where both were seen with a period of overlap on analysis of the EPG data. An example of this can be seen in Figure 8.4. During closure for the target bilabial stop in 'book', the subject makes both velar and alveolar EPG contacts. Although full closure is not made for the velar, this is considered spatially normal for a velar plosive. A period of double articulation can

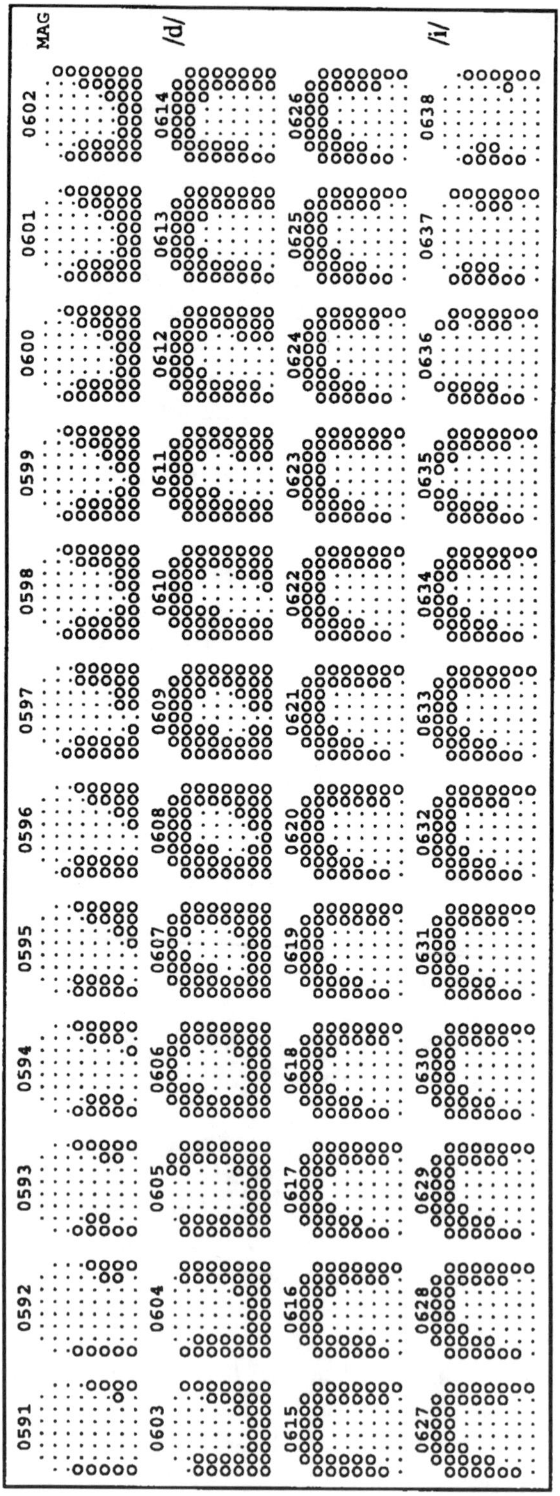

Figure 8.3: WI (word initial) misdirected velar gesture produced by BT (an apraxic speaker) during production of the word 'deer' variously transcribed as [gdiə] or [diə]. Taken from Hardcastle et al. 1985 (p.258)

be seen from frames 148 to 150 inclusive. The velar and alveolar contacts are released prior to the bilabial plosive, which is presumably why they are undetected through auditory analysis. Release of the bilabial plosive can be seen in Figure 8.5, which indicates the temporal position of the velar and alveolar lingual palatal contacts during the bilabial closure.

Wood (1997) noted that two of the aphasic speakers seemed to use MAGs as a strategy to achieve the correct target articulation. During repetition tasks, MU (Broca's aphasic with AOS) frequently produced an alveolar gesture in addition to the target velar plosive. The alveolar was produced prior to the velar in eight out of 12 productions of 'clock' and six out of 12 attempts at 'kitkat'. It seemed that the velar target was often triggered by the production of an alveolar MAG. Figure 8.6 shows an example of this 'triggering' phenomenon. For IE (conduction aphasic), if an alveolar MAG was detected during the production of a target velar, the velar was consistently produced first, followed by the MAG. Furthermore, the timing of this triggering was consistent over successive repetitions. Therefore the velar/alveolar sequence appeared to be a coordinated structure. This pattern is the reverse of the spatial sequencing noted for MU.

Howard (1998), in her case study of a patient with severe acquired apraxia of speech, noted an almost complete absence of MAGs. However, she notes that these began to appear when velars were targeted and introduced during EPG therapy.

These MAGs are felt to be important since they may provide valuable information regarding the source of the error. In particular, analysis of the lingual palatal contact patterns and the relationship that the misdirected gesture holds with other target phonemes in the word may help in identifying whether the error is linguistic or motoric in origin, or indeed, both. If the spatial configuration of the MAG is similar to the target sound produced elsewhere then the MAG may be considered an error in phonemic selection (Hardcastle and Edwards, 1992).

Errors in sequencing and selection versus distortions

Hardcastle et al. (1985), in their study investigating articulatory and voicing characteristics of two adult dysarthric and one adult apraxic speaker, identified characteristics which not only distinguished the two conditions as separate neurogenic disorders but also found similarities between them. Whereas the dysarthric errors were mostly distortions of the target configuration, the apraxic speech was characterized primarily by errors of sequencing and selection. However, both demonstrated spatial and temporal variability in their attempts at the targets, but these were more prominent in the speech of the apraxic. However, Southwood et al. (1997) noted articulatory undershoots, often associated with dysarthria, in the speech of their apraxic subject. Howard's (1998) investigation of a patient with severe acquired apraxia of speech identified both distortions and seriation difficulties.

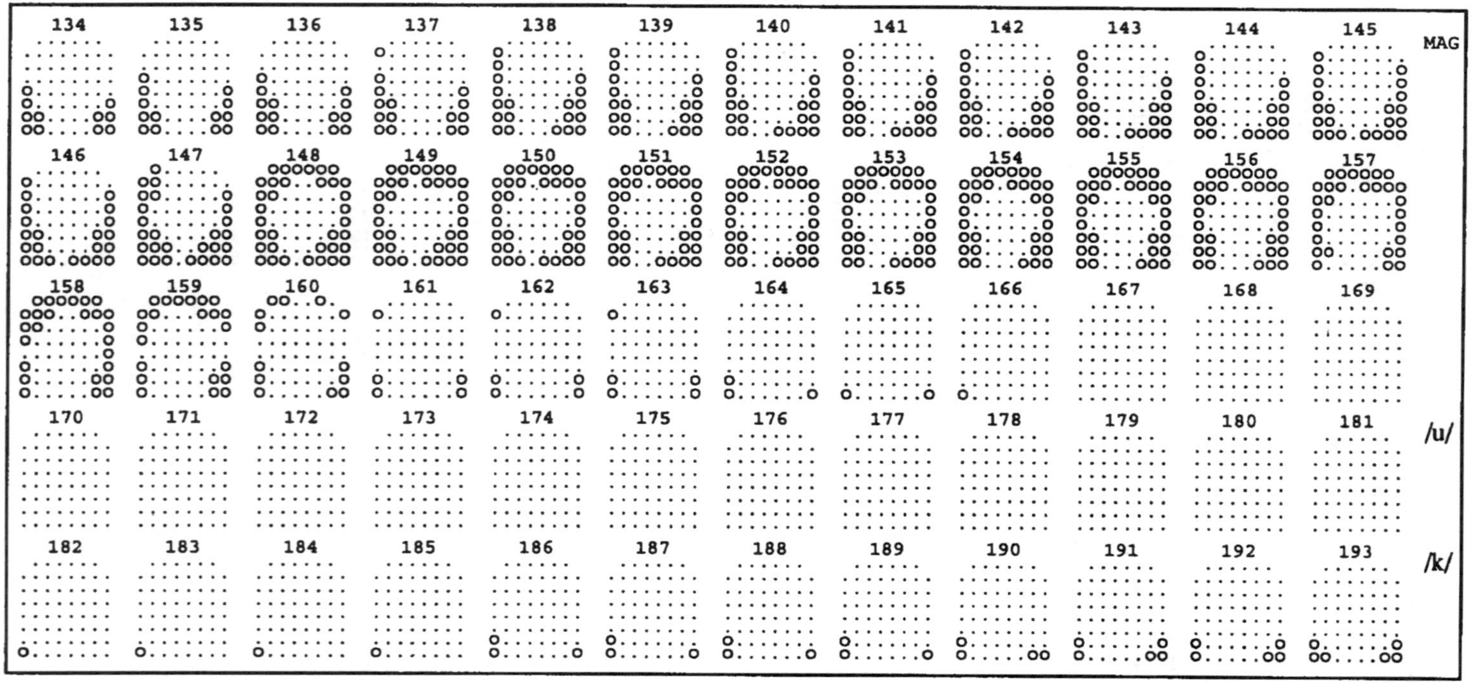

Figure 8.4: EPG print-out of the word 'book' produced by IE (a conduction aphasic). The word was heard as [ðə buk].

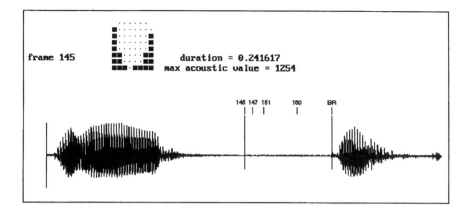

Figure 8.5: Acoustic waveform of the word 'book' produced by IE (a conduction aphasic). Frames corresponding to the EPG print-out are shown in Figure 8.4. The point of bilabial release, as detected from the acoustic signal, is marked BR.

Manner and place of production

The articulatory errors that have been identified by analysis of EPG in acquired neurogenic speech disorders have not been restricted to a single manner or place of articulation (Hardcastle et al., 1985; Hardcastle, 1987; Edwards and Miller, 1989; Hardcastle and Edwards, 1992; Wood, 1997). However, the frequency of the error type has varied between studies but is probably a direct result of methodological differences.

Disturbed temporal overlap in stop-stop sequences

Ingram and Hardcastle (1990) looked specifically at the coarticulatory abilities of a single apraxic and two control speakers. Their study involved the perceptual investigation of coarticulatory effects in conjunction with EPG and spectrographic analysis of the speech signal. The perceptual analysis noted less consistency in listeners' responses made from apraxic speech compared with the controls, and anticipatory coarticulation was not so strongly perceived in the apraxic speech. The EPG analysis suggested that the apraxic speaker avoided temporal overlap and showed abnormally long latencies between the two consonant gestures in words such as 'kitkat', 'tickling' and so on. In addition, Ingram and Hardcastle (1990) noted abnormal EPG patterns (for example, double alveolar/velar articulations during the word initial /t/ in 'tickling') which were not identified through perceptual auditory analysis. They suggested that these gestures were not identified because they had no acoustic consequences.

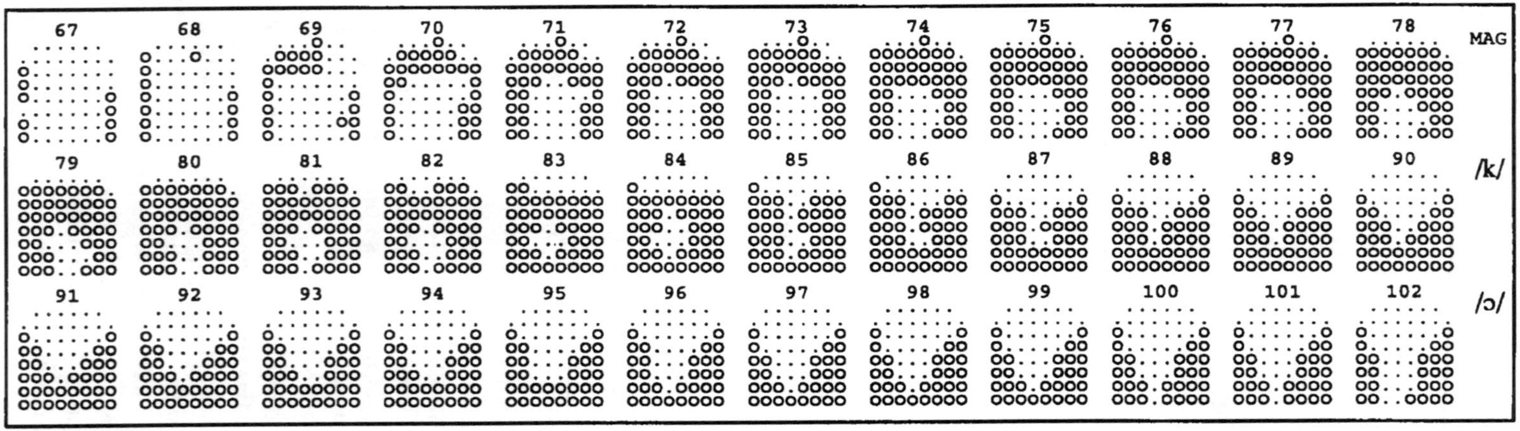

Figure 8.6: EPG print-out of the WI alveolar MAG and velar target in 'clock' produced by MU (Broca's aphasic with AOS). Phonetic transcription for this production was [ðə xɪɔk].

A lack of temporal overlap in consonant sequences was identified by Edwards and Miller (1989) and Hardcastle and Edwards (1992). The former study involved a single speaker whose lingual palatal contact patterns were also analysed by Hardcastle and Edwards (1992). Seriation problems were noted for all four apraxic speakers. These frequently took the form of abnormally long latencies between the alveolar and velar or velar and alveolar sequences, for example the word initial /kl/ sequence in 'clock' or the word medial /tk/ sequence in 'kitkat'. One subject demonstrated difficulty in alveolar/velar sequences but did not demonstrate abnormally long latencies during the production of velar/alveolar sequences. In addition to transitional timing deficits, Hardcastle and Edwards (1992) also noted errors in the sequencing of the target phonemes, which often resulted in reversal in the ordering of the two gestures, for example, during production of 'catkin' the /k/ gesture in the word medial sequence preceded the /t/ gesture.

Wood (1997) analysed in detail stop-stop consonant sequences during production of the word 'clock' and 'kitkat' 10 times by nine aphasic speakers and 10 normal speakers, each word preceded by the indefinite article. Productions of the /kl/ sequences were compared with patterns previously identified by Hardcastle (1985) from the speech of non-neurogenically impaired adults.

The aphasics (with and without AOS) were generally more variable in their sequencing patterns than normal speakers. However, the mean duration between stop-stop gestures in 'clock' when the velar was released prior to the onset of the tongue tip/blade movement (see Hardcastle, 1985) were comparable. For normal subjects the mean duration was 80 milliseconds, compared with 90 milliseconds for aphasic productions. Graphical displays were constructed to highlight the differences in stop-stop sequencing patterns between the aphasic speakers and the control speakers (see Figures 8.7–8.10).

Figure 8.7 (MU, Broca's with AOS) and Figure 8.8 (CR, Broca's without AOS) highlight the aphasic speakers' productions compared with the normal speakers (Figures 8.9 and 8.10). MU is consistent inasmuch as he omits the lateral approximant in all productions (see Figure 8.7). For seven repetitions a misdirected alveolar articulation was noted, which was typical of a stop closure for this subject. These MAGs vary considerably in their length (compare R5 at 70 ms with R2 at 570 ms). They also differ with regard to the sequencing of the velar closure. Four of the MAGs are articulated and released prior to the velar closure (R1, R3, R4 and R5), one is released at the point of velar closure (R2), and one commences prior to velar closure and overlaps briefly with it (R6). R9 shows a different pattern again. R7 and R8 show a single velar articulation. Durations of the velar articulation over the 10 repetitions vary considerably (170–360 ms) with a standard deviation of 79.554, which was much greater than that calculated for the control speakers.

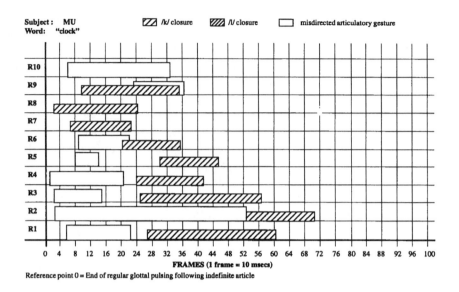

Figure 8.7: Sequencing of /kl/ in clock produced by MU.

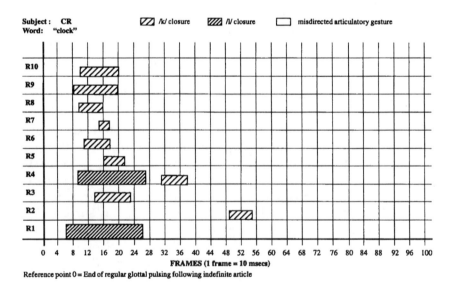

Figure 8.8: Sequencing of /kl/ in clock produced by CR.

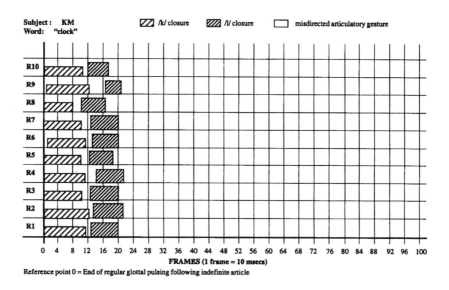

Figure 8.9: Sequencing of /kl/ in clock produced by KM.

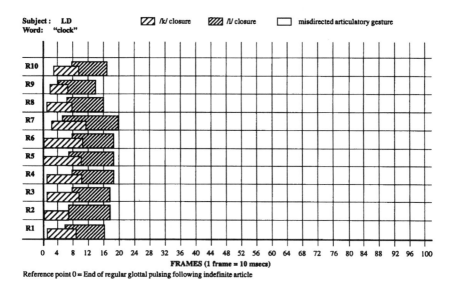

Figure 8.10: Sequencing of /kl/ in clock produced by LD.

Figure 8.8 (CR) clearly identifies the intra-subject variability of both the duration of individual phonemes and the sequencing and production of these. CR produced a single phoneme instead of a cluster for nine out of the 10 repetitions. Eight of these were single velar articulations and one was a single lateral articulation. In R4 CR produced both velar and alveolar lingual/palatal contacts but these were in the reverse order to the target sequence. The /l/ was articulated and released prior to the velar closure. This was considered to be a lateral approximant and not an MAG since its spatial appearance was similar to a target /l/ for this subject. The durations of the individual repetitions are also variable. The productions seem to become more consistent with time. R6 to R10 seem more uniform, with similar points for start and finish. The overall impression from Figure 8.8 is that CR produces much greater intra-subject variability than any of the control subjects, especially with regard to the production and sequencing of individual gestures.

In contrast, the normal subjects show very little variation in their productions (see Figures 8.9 and 8.10). In Figure 8.9 the velar gesture is released consistently prior to alveolar closure. In contrast, Figure 8.10 shows temporal overlap of the two gestures. Both patterns are considered normal and differences in timing are possibly related to regional variations between the speakers.

The word medial /tk/ sequence in 'kitkat' also highlighted differences between aphasic speakers and normal speakers. Whereas the normal speakers frequently assimilated the /t/ to the velar place of articulation (47% of productions) this was evident in only 8.9% of aphasic productions. The most common sequencing pattern produced by the aphasic speakers was the release of the alveolar closure prior to the /k/ closure (54% of productions). This pattern was seen in only 16% of normal speakers' repetitions. Conduction and anomic aphasics favoured this pattern (92% of productions). The most common /tk/ sequencing pattern for normal speakers (involving assimilation) can be seen in Figure 8.11 and, for aphasics, in Figure 8.12.

Southwood et al. (1997) were interested in the coarticulation of CV sequences for one apraxic and one normal speaker. Using gated speech stimuli listeners had to judge which vowel, /ɑ,æ, i, ɪ, u, ʊ/, followed either a voiced bilabial plosive or a voiceless palatal fricative. They noted delayed and distorted coarticulatory gestures which were further disturbed when speaking rate was altered. The appropriate articulatory configurations were reached later in the vowel compared with normal speakers.

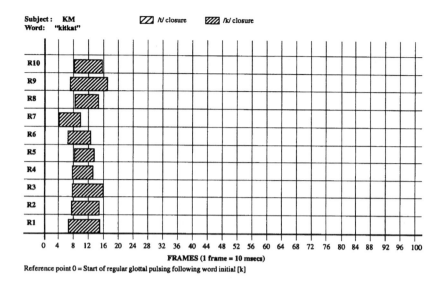

Figure 8.11: Sequencing of /tk/ in 'kitkat' produced by KM.

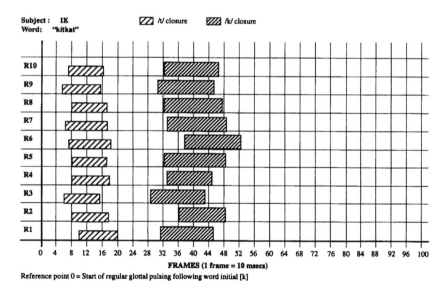

Figure 8.12: Sequencing of /tk/ in 'kitkat' produced by IE.

Syllable segregation

Through studying the non-speech oral movements of a patient with severe acquired apraxia of speech (AD), Howard (1998) identified abnormal movement patterns. AD was taught to produce velar closures through visual feedback from EPG and to alternate between front and back lingual palatal closures. While training AD, Howard noticed that the alternating movements were unlike a normal speaker, who used the lateral margins of the tongue as a pivot between front and back closures (as in Figure 8.13). In contrast AD alternated an alveolar closure with a distorted back closure but there appeared to be no consistent involvement of the lateral margins (see Figure 8.14).

These findings were taken to suggest that each closure and release sequence was produced in isolation. Since this segregation of movement mirrored AD's production of CV syllable gestures, Howard suggests that syllable segregation is not a compensatory strategy used in speech production to assist speech intelligibility. Instead she argues that it is a 'product of a specific motor constraint, rather than being compensatory in nature' (1998: 386).

Treatment of acquired neurogenic speech disorders using EPG

Principles of EPG therapy

Therapy that employs visual feedback enables the client to visualize their speech output. The procedure involves discussing with the client the target speech pattern and highlighting the speech errors. The client then practises the target articulation, modifying it until it matches the visual display.

EPG has been used successfully in therapy for clients with acquired neurogenic speech disorders who are experiencing articulation difficulties, specifically lingual palatal placement abnormalities and/or lingual dynamics. In choosing a client for EPG therapy a number of factors must be taken into consideration. These include:

- aetiological factors, for example, sensory loss;
- psychological factors such as the client's cognitive abilities and motivation;
- physical and physiological factors including attention span, levels of fatigue and general health;
- the client's awareness of their difficulties, auditory discrimination and linguistic difficulties;
- personal factors such as their emotional state and expectations of EPG therapy.

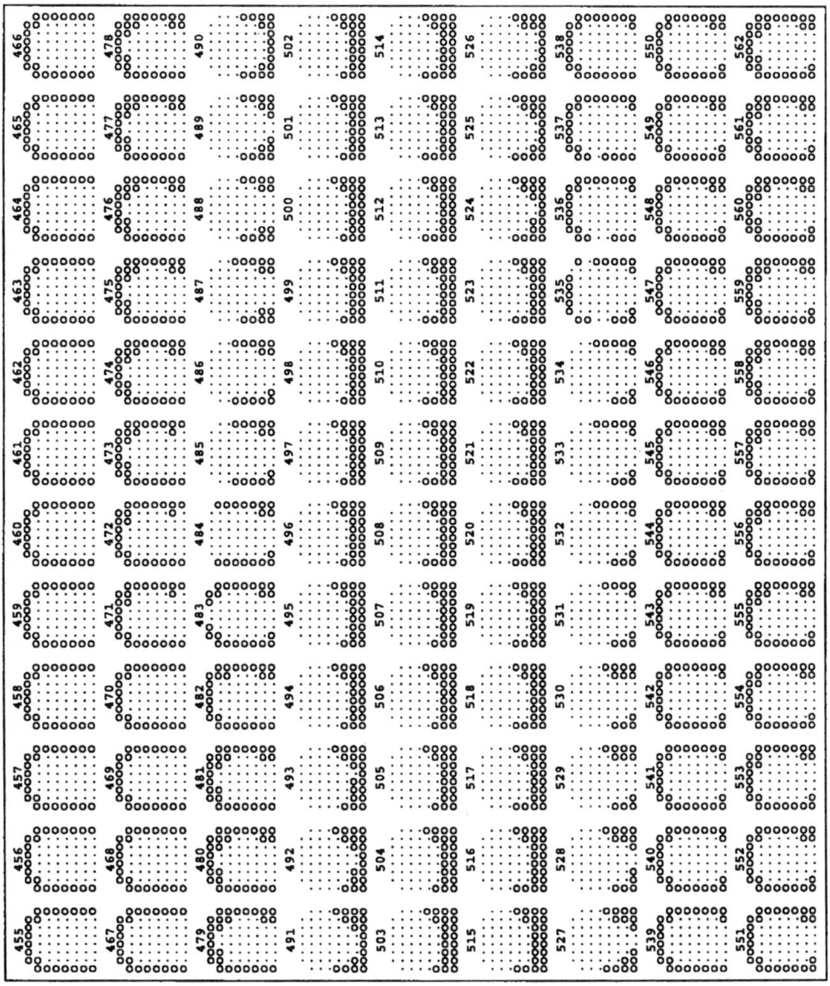

Figure 8.13: Lingual palatal contact patterns for a normal speaker producing front–back alternating movements (taken from Howard, 1998).

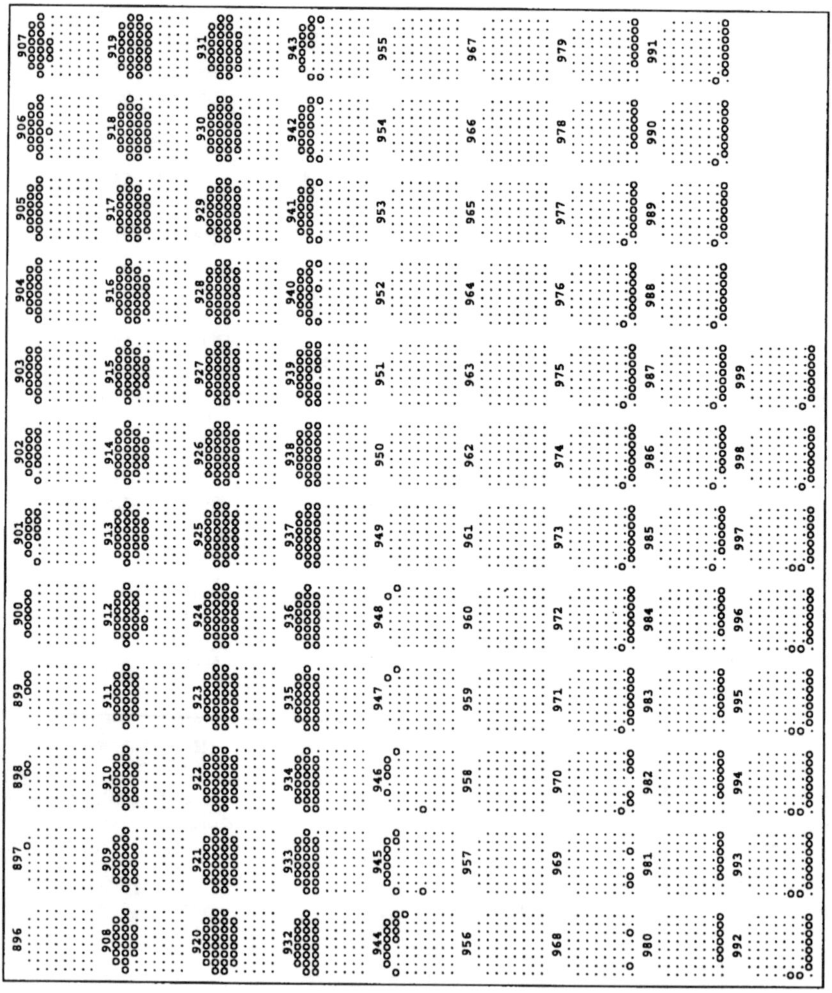

Figure 8.14: AD's lingual palatal contact patterns for front–back alternating movements (taken from Howard, 1998).

For a more detailed discussion of these issues the reader is directed to Morgan Barry (1989) and Hardcastle, Gibbon and Jones (1991).

Stages in EPG therapy

EPG therapy involves three broad stages: a demonstration phase, a monitoring phase and a carry-over phase. During the demonstration phase the relationship of the tongue with the hard palate and the acoustic consequence must be demonstrated and explained. The visual display on the EPG monitor must be linked to the tongue and hard palate. Once this has been comprehended, the differences between correct and incorrect patterns can be explained. Following this stage the client is encouraged to learn new motor skills in a stepwise fashion using a target configuration produced by the clinician and the real-time display of the client's patterns. Initially, the clinician encourages the client to build an awareness of motor patterns and gross movements, for example, front–back contrasts. Then, specific articulatory postures are targeted, often without voicing or air stream to begin with. Next, the targeted sound is produced in differing vowel contexts before moving on to phonemic contrasts, which often involve minimal pairs. Once this has been mastered the client attempts more complex phonetic contrasts, for example clusters, phrases and conversational speech. During the carry-over phase the client has to recall the new motor patterns that he has learned without the visual feedback and the palate is removed. For more details on therapeutic procedures the reader is directed to Hardcastle et al. (1991) and Hardcastle and Gibbon (1997).

EPG therapy in adults with acquired neurogenic speech disorders

Morgan Barry (1989), Howard and Varley (1995) and Howard (1998) have all reported individual case studies involving EPG therapy with clients with apraxia of speech. Goldstein et al. (1994) used combined EPG and palatal lift to improve the speech of a client with acquired dysarthria.

Morgan Barry (1989) describes one subject (Mr T) with mild to moderate dyspraxia. His speech was characterized by hesitations and dysfluencies and sound searching behaviours were evident both acoustically and from analysis of the EPG contact patterns. The aim of the intervention was for the client to develop visual kinaesthetic awareness, which would reduce the sound searching behaviours. In her evaluation of the therapy, Morgan Barry noted that Mr T was 'able to use the instrumentation in conjunction with slowed speech in order to monitor movements and increase kinaesthetic awareness' (1989: 90).

Howard and Varley (1995) and Howard (1998) report on a patient (AD) with severe acquired apraxia of speech. Following assessment using EPG they noted that the tip/blade of the tongue appeared to be an active and separate articulator from the tongue body, but that the tongue body had only a secondary role. There was little evidence of palatal and velar closures independent of the alveolar region. It was felt that AD had a sensory-perceptual impairment since he reported abnormalities in oral sensation and was unable to monitor his tongue position and movements. Therefore the authors predicted that EPG would provide an alternative system of feedback to assist AD in monitoring his speech.

Initially, therapy concentrated on introducing finer and more differentiated control of the tongue and distinguishing front and back contrasts before focusing on speech sounds. Howard and Varley (1995) and Howard (1998) noted that AD produced different non-speech front closure patterns than he did alveolar closure during speech production (/d,dj,n,nj/). The non-speech patterns were similar to a normal alveolar lateral approximant (/l/) (see Figure 8.15a) compared with the alveolar closures that resembled normal alveolar plosives (see Figure 8.15b). They used this distinction to introduce the contrast between /d/ and /l/ and to try to bring this under voluntary control. They initially taught the contrasts as silent steady-state patterns before progressing on to nonsense words and minimal pairs. AD became proficient at producing /l/, which was auditorily acceptable. However, production of /d/ was variable and often indistinguishable from /l/. Detailed analysis of the EPG patterns revealed that the approach and release phases of the /d/ were often inappropriate even when the steady-state closure phase was considered normal. Instead of the contacts for the alveolar plosive building from the back of the palate and spreading to the front as would be expected in the approach phase and releasing from front to back (Figure 8.16), AD produced the reverse of this sequence (Figure 8.17). The contacts were initially made in the alveolar region and these spread backwards to include the lateral seals, and the release started from the back and spread forwards. Once the correct dynamic patterns had been demonstrated and achieved, more complex structures were introduced, for example 'lad', 'ladder' and 'doll', 'dollar'. What is interesting is that sequences where the second consonant built on lingual palatal contacts made for the first consonant ('lad', 'ladder') were less problematic than the reverse when contacts had to be suppressed ('doll', 'dollar').

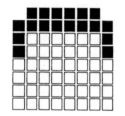

Figure 8.15a: Normal lingual palatal contacts for lateral approximant /l/.

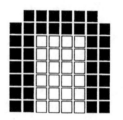

Figure 8.15b: Normal lingual palatal contacts for alveolar plosive /d/.

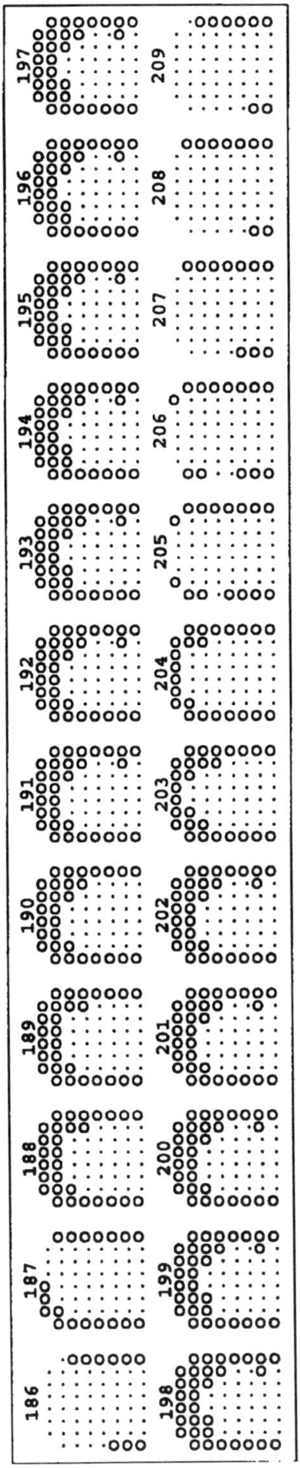

Figure 8.16: Normal speaker's lingual palatal contact patterns for /d/ (taken from Howard and Varley, 1995).

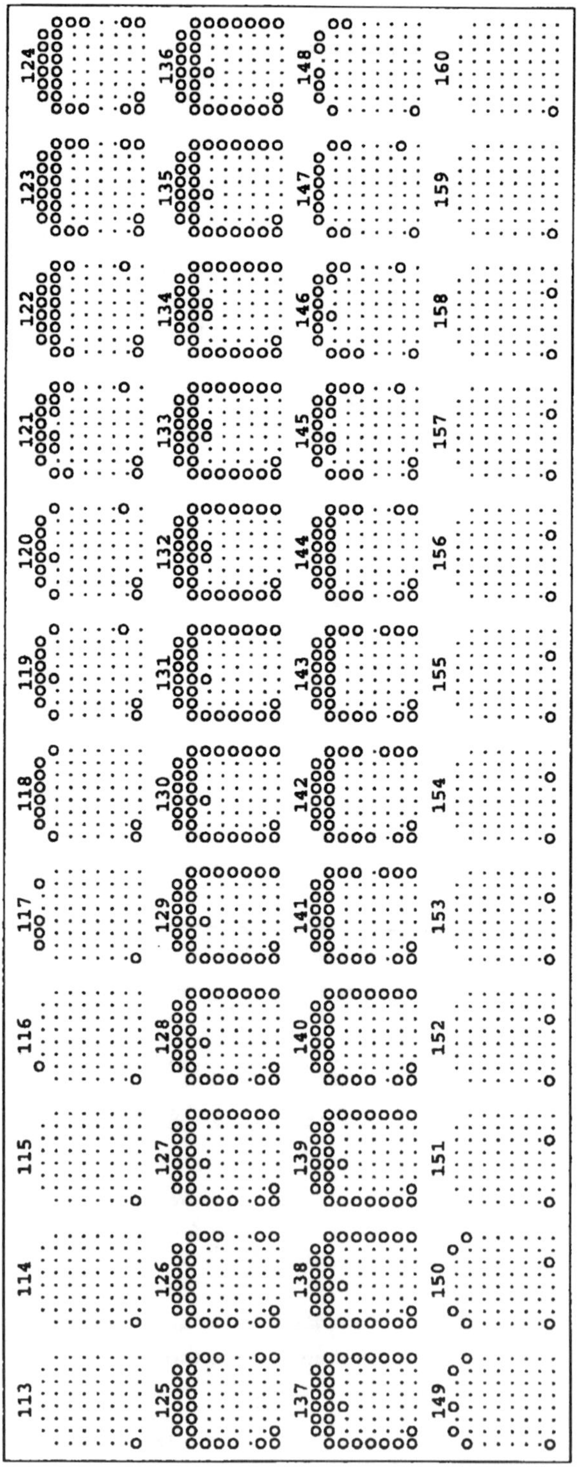

Figure 8.17: AD's abnormal approach and release phase for /d/ (taken from Howard and Varley, 1995).

Once the above contrast had been mastered, articulations involving the velar portion of the palate were introduced. AD's articulations were then considered to be more usual for an apraxic speaker with evidence of lingual groping emerging. In their conclusion, Howard and Varley state that: 'It cannot be assumed that in achieving target steady-state lingual strictures a speaker with apraxia will take the same articulatory route as a normal speaker' (1995: 255).

Goldstein et al. (1994) reported on the therapeutic intervention in a case of severe dysarthria following a closed head injury combining palatal lift with EPG feedback. The most prominent feature of the subject's speech was a severe velopharnygeal incompetence. Additionally, they described a deficit in lingual control which manifested itself in the form of imprecise or vowel-like consonants. Goldstein et al. (1994) suggested that this was indicative of undershooting of labial and lingual movements. They also noted occasional overshooting of tongue movements which resulted in click-like sounds and reduced rates during rapid syllable repetition.

Therapy was divided into four phases: preparatory phase, palatal lift phase, EPG-feedback training, and consolidation and individual communicative skill training. The EPG phase involved practising non-speech movements prior to alveolar, palatal and velar consonants.

Goldstein et al. report many articulatory changes as a result of the EPG feedback. They noticed a consistent advancement of the tongue and a closer, more normal constriction pattern during production of alveolar fricatives. They conclude that the changes 'suggest that he has learnt to exploit kinaesthetic and acoustic sources of feedback and interpret them in terms of appropriate lingual adjustments' (1994: 211).

Summary of assessment and therapy using EPG

While the assessment and treatment of acquired neurogenic speech disorders using EPG have been limited to a few case studies, the value of the instrumental technique cannot be denied. Direct assessment of lingual palatal contacts in real time has identified many errors (for example, MAGs and errors in sequencing and timing) which are inaudible. In her study, Wood made a distinction between 'pure' substitutions, which she defined as 'errors where the lingual/palatal contact patterns confirmed the auditory impression' (1997: 105) and auditorily perceived substitutions, where lingual/palatal contact patterns were not detected on auditory analysis but were evident from analysis of the EPG data. Analysis of the EPG data revealed that 25% of the perceived substitutions showed lingual palatal contact patterns that were not detected through auditory analysis and were therefore not 'pure' substitutions. These observations have important implications for understanding the level of impairment, the subsequent development of models of speech production and the development of appropriate and efficacious therapeutic intervention programmes. Clearly, the additional visual feedback provided by EPG therapy enabled the subjects in the studies quoted above to understand their errors and to modify their speech production. The visual feedback provided an alternative means by which neurogenically impaired speakers could monitor their own speech and make necessary adjustments.

Conclusion

In this chapter we have outlined the wide range of instrumental techniques available for use in various aspects of assessment and treatment of acquired neurogenic disorders. As we indicated, the advantages of instrumental analysis over traditional auditory-based judgements are clear, but there are relatively few techniques that satisfy all the prerequisites for clinical use. Many are still in prototype form and are too expensive for the average clinic or require elaborate setting up and preparation of the subject. We have chosen to concentrate on EPG as it is non-invasive, relatively inexpensive and provides unique quantitative and qualitative data on one aspect of lingual movement. This has proven to have been of considerable clinical relevance in areas such as differential diagnosis. Although there have been relatively few case studies using EPG as a biofeedback technique in this client group, initial results have been promising and we can expect an expansion in this area of activity as EPG devices become more widely available. The widespread use of EPG has been considerably boosted recently by the development of a cheaper, therapy-only device (PTU – Portable Training Unit) based on an LED display of tongue-palate contacts. This new device has been successfully trialled recently in the project CLEFTNET involving cleft palate clients throughout Scotland.

Notes

1. See discussion in Stevens (1997) and Hardcastle and Marchal (1990).
2. See, for example, Weismer (1984a, 1984b), Orlikoff and Baken (1993) and Kent and Read (1992).
3. For example, the laryngograph – see descriptions in Abberton and Fourcin (1997), Fourcin and Abberton (1971) and Motta et al. (1990).
4. See survey in Thompson-Ward and Murdoch (1998).
5. Further discussions can be found in Blair and Smith (1986) and Wohlert and Goffman (1994).

References

Abberton E, Fourcin A (1997). Electrolaryngography. In Ball MJ, Code C (eds) Instrumental Clinical Phonetics. London: Whurr, pp.119–48.

Ackermann H, Gröne BF, Hoch G, Schönle PW (1993). Speech freezing in Parkinson's disease: a kinematic analysis of orofacial movements by means of electromagnetic articulography. Folio Phoniatrica 45: 84–9.

Amorosa H, Benda V, Von Wagner E, Keck A (1985). Transcribing phonetic detail in the speech of unintelligible children: a comparison of procedures. British Journal of Disorders of Communication 20: 281–7.

Anthony J, Hewlett N (1984). Aerometry. In Code C, Ball M (eds) Experimental Clinical Phonetics. London: Croom Helm, pp.79–106.

Baer T, Gore J, Gracco V, Nye P (1991). Analysis of vocal tract shape and dimensions using magnetic resonance imaging: vowels. Journal of Acoustical Society of America 90: 799–828.

Baken RJ (1987). Clinical Measurement of Speech and Voice. Boston, MA: College Hill.

Baken RJ, Orlikoff RF (2nd Edition, in press). Clinical Measurements of Speech and Voice. San Diego, CA: Singular.

Ball MJ (1984). X-ray techniques. In Code C, Ball M (eds) Experimental Clinical Phonetics. London: Croom Helm, pp.107–28.

Ball MJ (1991). Recent developments in the transcription of non-normal speech. Journal of Communication Disorders 25: 59–78.

Ball MJ, Code C (1997). Instrumental Clinical Phonetics. London: Whurr.

Ball MJ, Gröne B (1997). Imaging techniques. In Ball MJ, Code C (eds) Instrumental Clinical Phonetics. London: Whurr, pp.194–227.

Barlow SM, Cole KJ, Abbs JH (1983). A new head-mounted lip-jaw movement transduction system for the study of motor speech disorders. Journal of Speech and Hearing Disorders 26: 283–8.

Basmajian JV (1979). Biofeedback – Principles and Practice for Clinicians. Baltimore, MD: Williams and Wilkins.

Basmajian JV, De Luca CJ (1985). Muscles Alive: Their Functions Revealed by Electromyography (5th Edition). Baltimore, MD: Williams and Wilkins.

Blair C, Smith A (1986). EMG recording in human lip muscles: can single muscles be isolated? Journal of Speech and Hearing Research 29: 256–66.

Blumstein S (1973). A Phonological Investigation of Aphasic Speech. The Hague: Mouton & Co.

Branderud P (1985). Movetrack – a movement tracking system. Proceedings of the French Swedish Symposium on Speech. 22–4 April 1985, Grenoble, GALF, 113–22.

Buckingham HW, Yule G (1987). Phonetic false evaluation: theoretical and clinical aspects. Clinical Linguistics and Phonetics 1: 113–25.

Canter GJ, Trost JE, Burns MS (1985). Contrasting speech patterns in apraxia of speech and phonemic paraphasia. Brain and Language 24: 204–22.

Cavallo SA, Baken RJ (1985). Prephonatory laryngeal and chest wall dynamics. Journal of Speech and Hearing Research 28: 79–87.

Coleman RF (1983). Instrumental analysis of voice disorders. Seminars in Speech and Language 4: 205–15.

Dagenais PA, Critz-Crosby P (1992). Comparing tongue positioning by normal hearing and hearing impaired children during vowel production. Journal of Speech and Hearing Research 35: 35–44.

Dalston RM (1982). Photodetector assessment of velopharygeal function. Cleft Palate Journal 19: 1–8.

Dicenta M, Oliveras J (1976). La Xeroradiología Lareíngea. Acta Otorinolaringologica Española 27: 99–106.

Duckworth M, Allen G, Hardcastle WH, Ball M (1990). Extensions to the International Phonetic Alphabet for the transcription of atypical speech. Clinical Linguistics and Phonetics 4: 273–80.

Dworkin JP, Aronson AE (1986). Tongue strength and alternate motion rates in normal and dysarthric speakers. Journal of Communication Disorders 19: 115–32.

Edwards S, Miller N (1989). Using EPG to investigate speech errors and motor agility in a dyspraxic patient. Clinical Linguistics and Phonetics 3(1): 111–26.

Ellis RE, Flack FC, Curle HJ, Selley WG (1978). A system for the assessment of airflow during speech. British Journal of Disorders of Communication 13: 31–40.

Farmer A (1997). Spectography. In Code C, Ball M (eds) Instrumental Clinical Phonetics. London: Whurr, pp.21–40.

Farnetani E, Provaglio A (1991). Assessing variability of lingual consonants in Italian. Quaderni del Centro di Studio per le Ricerche di Fonetica del CNR X: 117–45.

Fletcher SG (1970). Theory and instrumentation for quantitative measurement of nasality. Cleft Palate Journal 7: 601–9.

Forrest K, Adams S, McNeil MR, Southwood H (1991). Kinematic electromyographic, and perceptual evaluation of speech apraxia, conduction aphasia, ataxic dysarthria and normal speech production. In Moore CA, Yorkston KM, Beukelman DR (eds) Dysarthria and Apraxia of Speech. Baltimore, MD: Brookes, pp.147–71.

Fourcin AJ, Abberton E (1971). First applications of a new laryngograph. Medical and Biological Illustration 21: 172–82.

Fujimura O, Erickson D (1997). Acoustic phonetics. In Hardcastle WJ, Laver J (eds) Instrumental Clinical Phonetics. Oxford: Blackwell, pp.61–115.

Gentil M, Moore WH (1997). Electromyography. In Ball MJ, Code C (eds) Instrumental Clinical Phonetics. London: Whurr, pp.64–86.

Gerratt BR, Till JA, Rosenbek JC, Wertz RT, Boysen AE (1991). Use and perceived value of perceptual and instrumental measures in dysarthria management. In Moore CA, Yorkston KM, Beukelman DR (eds) Dysarthria and Apraxia of Speech. Baltimore, MD: Brookes, pp.77–93.

Goldstein P, Ziegler W, Vogel M, Hoole P (1994). Combined palatal-lift and EPG-feedback therapy in dysarthria: a case study. Clinical Linguistics and Phonetics 8(3): 201–18.

Hardcastle WJ (1985). Some phonetic and syntactic constraints on lingual co-articulation during /kl/ sequences. Speech Communication 4: 247–63.

Hardcastle WJ (1987). Electropalatographic study of articulation disorders in verbal dyspraxia. In Ryalls J (ed.) Phonetic Approaches to Speech Production in Aphasia and Related Disorders. San Diego, CA: College Hill, pp.113–36.

Hardcastle WJ, Edwards S (1992). EPG-based description of apraxic speech errors. In Kent R (ed.) Intelligibility in Speech Disorders. Amsterdam/Philadelphia, PA: John Benjamins, pp.287–328.

Hardcastle WJ, Gibbon F (1997). Electropalatography and its clinical applications. In Ball MJ, Code C (eds) Instrumental Clinical Phonetics. London: Whurr, pp.149–93.

Hardcastle WJ, Gibbon FE, Jones W (1991). Visual display of tongue-palate contact: electropalatography in the assessment and remediation of speech disorders. British Journal of Disorders of Communication 26: 41–74.

Hardcastle WJ, Laver J (eds) (1997) The Handbook of Phonetic Sciences. Oxford: Blackwell.

Hardcastle WJ, Marchal A (eds) (1990) Speech Production and Speech Modelling. Dordrecht: Kluwer.

Hardcastle WJ, Morgan Barry RA, Clark CJ (1985). Articulatory and voicing characteristics of adult dysarthric and verbal dyspraxic speakers: an instrumental study. British Journal of Disorders of Communication 20: 249–70.

Harrington J (1986). The Phonetic Analysis of Stuttering. Unpublished PhD dissertation, University of Cambridge.

Hinton VA, Luschei ES (1992). Validation of a modern miniature transducer for measurement of interlabial contact pressures during speech. Journal of Speech and Hearing Research 35: 245–51.

Hirose H, Kiritani S, Ushijima T, Sawashima M (1978). Analysis of abnormal articulatory dynamics in two dysarthric patients. Journal of Speech and Hearing Disorders 43: 96–105.

Hirose H, Kiritani S, Ushijima T, Yoshioka H, Sawashima M (1981). Patterns of dysarthric movements in patients with Parkinsonism. Folia Phoniatrica 33: 204–15.

Hixon TJ, Putnam AH, and Sharp JT (1983). Speech production with flaccid paralysis of the rib cage, diaphragm and abdomen. Journal of Speech and Hearing Disorders 48: 315–27.

Hoodin RB, Gilbert HR (1989). Nasal airflows in Parkinsonian speakers. Journal of Communication Disorders 22: 169–80.

Hoole P, Kühnert B, Mooshammer T, Tillmann HG (eds) (1993). Proceedings of the ACCOR Workshop on Electromagnetic Articulography in Phonetic Research. Forschungsberichte des Instituts für Phonetik und Sprachliche Kommunikation der Universität München (FIPKM) 31.

Horiguchi S, Bell-Berti F (1987). The Velotrace: a device for monitoring velar position. Cleft Palate Journal 24: 104–11.

Horii Y (1983). An accelerometric measure as a physical correlate of perceived hypernasality in speech. Journal of Speech and Hearing Research 26: 476–80.

Howard S (1998). Phonetic constraints on phonological systems: combining perceptual and instrumental analysis in the investigation of speech disorders (Volume 1). Unpublished PhD dissertation, University of Sheffield.

Howard S, Varley R (1995). Using electropalatography to treat severe acquired apraxia of speech. European Journal of Disorders of Communication 30(2): 246–55.

Howard S, Varley R (1996). Perceptual, electropalatographic and acoustic analysis of a case of severe acquired apraxia of speech. In Powell TW (ed.) Pathologies of Speech and Language: Contributions of Clinical Phonetics and Linguistics. New Orleans, LA: ICPLA, pp.237–45.

Huffman AL (1978). Biofeedback treatment of orofacial dysfunction: a preliminary study. American Journal of Occupational Therapy 32: 149–54.

Ingram J, Hardcastle WJ (1990). Perceptual, acoustic and electropalatographic evaluation of coarticulation effects in apraxic speech. In Seidle R (ed.) Proceedings of 3rd Australian International Conference on Speech Science and Technology. Canberra: Australian Speech Science and Technology Association, pp.110–15.

Itoh M, Sasanuma S (1984). Articulatory movements in apraxia of speech. In Rosenbek JC, McNeil M, Aronson A (eds) Apraxia of Speech. San Diego, CA: College Hill, pp.135–66.

Itoh M, Sasanuma S, Hirose H, Yoshioka H, Ushijima T (1980). Abnormal articulatory dynamics in a patient with apraxia of speech: X-ray microbeam observation. Brain and Language 11: 66–75.

Itoh M, Sasanuna S, Ushijima T (1979). Velar movements during speech in a patient with apraxia of speech. Brain and Language 7: 227–39.

Karling J, Lohmander A, De Serpa-Leitao A, Galyas K, Larson O (1985). NORAM: calibration and operational advice for measuring nasality in cleft palate patients. Scandinavian Journal of Plastic and Reconstructive Surgery 17: 33–50.

Katz W, Machetanz J, Orth U, Schönle P (1990). A kinematic analysis of anticipatory co-articulation in the speech of anterior aphasic subjects using electromagnetic articulography. Brain and Language 38: 555–75.

Keller E, Ostry DJ (1983). Computerised measurement of tongue closure movements with pulsed-echo ultrasound. Journal of Acoustical Society of America 73: 1309–15.

Kent R, Netsell R (1975). A case study of an ataxic dysarthric: cineradiographic and spectrographic observations. Journal of Speech and Hearing Disorders 40: 115–34.

Kent RD, Read C (1992). The Acoustic Analysis of Speech. San Diego, CA: Singular.

Kiritani S (1986). X-ray microbeam method for measurement of articulatory dynamics: techniques and results. Speech Communication 5: 119–40.

Koike Y, Perkins WH (1968). Application of a miniaturised pressure transducer for experimental speech research. Folia Phoniatrica 20: 360–8.

Künzel HJ (1977). Photoelektrische Untersuchung zur Velumhöhe bei Vokalen: erste Anvendung des Velographen. Phonetica 34: 352–70.

Lass NJ (1996). Principles of Experimental Phonetics. St. Louis, MO: Mosby.

Laver J (1994). Principles of Phonetics. Cambridge: Cambridge University Press.

Moore C (1992). The correspondence of vocal tract resonance with volumes obtained from magnetic resonance images. Journal of Speech and Hearing Research 35: 1009–23.

Morgan Barry R (1989). EPG from square one: an overview of electropalatography as an aid to therapy. Clinical Linguistics and Phonetics 3(1): 81–91.

Morgan Barry R (1995). Acquired dysarthria: a segmental phonological, prosodic and electropalatographic investigation of intelligibility. In Perkins M, Howard S (eds) Case Studies in Clinical Linguistics. London: Whurr, pp.181–211.

Motta G, Cesari U, Iengo M, Motta G (Jr) (1990). Clinical application of electroglottography. Folia Phoniatrica 42: 111–17.

Müller EM, Abbs JH (1979). Strain gauge transduction of lips and jaw motion in the midsagittal plane: experiment of a prototype system. Journal of the Acoustical Society of America 65: 481–6.

Murdoch B, Chenery H, Bowler S, Ingram J (1989). Respiratory function in Parkinson's subjects exhibiting a perceptible speech deficit: a kinematic and spirometric analysis. Journal of Speech and Hearing Disorders 54: 610–16.

Netsell R, Cleeland CS (1973). Modification of lip hypertonia in dysarthria using EMG feedback. Journal of Speech and Hearing Disorders 38: 131–40.

Netsell R, Lotz WK, Du Chane AS, Barlow SM (1991). Vocal tract aerodynamics during syllable productions: normative data and theoretical implications. Journal of Voice 5: 1–9.

Ohala JJ (1971). Monitoring soft palate movements in speech. Journal of the Acoustical Society of America 50: 140(A).

Orlikoff RF, Baken RJ (1993). Clinical Speech and Voice Measurement: Laboratory Exercises. San Diego, CA: Singular.

Perkell JS, Cohen MH, Svirsky MA, Matties ML, Garabieta I, Jackson MTT (1992). Electromagnetic midsagittal articulometer system for transducing speech articulatory movements. Journal of Acoustical Society of America 92: 3078–96.

Read C, Buder E, Kent RD (1990). Speech analysis systems: a survey. Journal of Speech and Hearing Research 33: 363–74.

Read C, Buder E, Kent RD (1992). Speech analysis systems: an evaluation. Journal of Speech and Hearing Research 35: 314–32.

Robin DA, Goel A, Somodi LB, Luschei ES (1992). Tongue strength and endurance: relation to highly skilled movements. Journal of Speech and Hearing Research 35: 1239–45.

Rothenberg M (1973). A new inverse-filtering technique for deriving the glottal air flow waveform during voicing. Journal of the Acoustical Society of America 53: 1632–45.

Rothenberg M (1977). Measurement of airflow in speech. Journal of Speech and Hearing Research 20: 155–76.

Rubow R (1984). Role of feedback, reinforcement and compliance on training and transfer in biofeedback-based rehabilitation of motor speech disorders. In McNeil MR, Rosenbek JC, Aronson AE (eds) The Dysarthrias: Physiology, Acoustics, Perception, Management. San Diego, CA: College Hill, pp.207–30.

Rubow RT, Rosenbek JC, Collins M, Celesia GC (1984). Reduction in hemifacial spasm and dysarthria following EMG biofeedback. Journal of Speech and Hearing Disorders 49: 26–33.

Schutte HK, Svec JG, Sram F (1997). Videokymography: research and clinical issues. Logopedics, Phoniatrics, Vocology 22(4): 152–6.

Schönle P, Gräbe K, Wenig P, Höhne J, Schrader J, Conrad B (1987). Electromagnetic articulography: use of alternative magnetic fields for tracking movements of multiple points inside and outside the vocal tract. Brain and Language 31: 26–35.

Seddoh SAK, Robin DA, Sim H, Hageman C, Moon JB, Folkins JW (1996). Speech timing in apraxia of speech versus conduction aphasia. Journal of Speech and Hearing Research 39: 590–603.

Skenes LL (1987). Durational changes of apraxic speakers. Journal of Communication Disorders 20: 61–71.

Southwood MH, Dagenais PA, Sutphin SM, Mertz Garcia J (1997). Coarticulation in apraxia of speech: a perceptual, acoustic and electropalatographic study. Clinical Linguistics and Phonetics 11(3): 179–203.

Sperry EE, Klich RJ (1992). Speech breathing in senescent and younger women during oral reading. Journal of Speech and Hearing Research 35: 1246–55.

Stevens KN (1997). Articulatory-acoustic-auditory relationships. In Hardcastle WJ, Laver J (eds) The Handbook of Phonetic Sciences. Oxford: Blackwell, pp.462–506.

Stevens KN, Kalikow DN, Willemain TR (1975). A miniature accelerometer for detecting glottal waveforms and nasalisation. Journal of Speech and Hearing Research 18: 594–9.

Stone M (1991). Imaging the tongue and vocal tract. British Journal of Disorders of Communication 26: 11–23.

Stone M (1996). Instrumentation for the study of speech physiology. In Lass NJ (ed.) Principles of Experimental Phonetics. St Louis, MO: Mosby, pp.495–524.

Stone M (1997). Investigating speech articulation. In Hardcastle WJ, Laver J (eds) Handbook of Phonetic Science. Oxford: Blackwell, pp.11–32.

Sugishita M, Konno K, Kabe S, Yunoki K, Togashi O, Kawamura M (1987). Electropalatographic analysis of apraxia of speech in a left-hander and in a right-hander. Brain 110: 1393–1417.

Thompson EC, Murdoch BE (1995). Disorders of nasality in subjects with upper motor neurone type dysarthria following cerebrovascular accident. Journal of Communication Disorders 28: 261–76.

Thompson-Ward EC, Murdoch BE (1998). Instrumental assessment of the speech mechanism. In Murdoch BE (ed.) Dysarthria: A Physiological Approach. Cheltenham: Stanley Thornes, pp.68–101.

Tuller B, Shao S, Kelso JAS (1990). An evaluation of an alternating magnetic field device for monitoring tongue movements. Journal of Acoustical Society of America 88: 674–9.

Vatikiotis-Bateson E, Ostry D (1995). An analysis of the dimensionality of jaw motion in speech. Journal of Phonetics 23: 101–19.

Vieregge WH (1978). Bemerkungen zum normal und gestört-sprachlichen kommunikator und das problem des transkription von gaumenspaltensprache. IFN–Proceedings (Institut Fonetik, Nijmegen) 2: 51–71.

Vieregge WH (1987). Probleme der phonetischen transkription. Zeitschrift für Dialektologie und Linguistik Beihefte 54: 5–55.

Warren DW (1996). Regulation of speech aerodynamics. In Lass NJ (ed.) Principles of Experimental Phonetics. St Louis, MO: Mosby, pp.46–92.

Warren DW, Dubois A (1964). A pressure-flow technique for measuring velopharyngeal orifice area during continuous speech. Cleft Palate Journal 1: 52–71.

Warren RM, Obusek CJ (1971). Speech perception and phonemic restoration. Perception and Psychophysics 9: 358–62.

Washino K, Kasai Y, Uchida Y, Takeda K (1981). Tongue movement during speech in a patient with apraxia of speech: a case study. In Peng FC (ed.) Current Issues in Neurolinguistics: A Japanese Contribution: Language Function and its Neural Mechanisms, Advances in Neurolinguistics, Proceedings of the 2nd ICU Conference of Neurolinguistics, Tokyo, pp.125–59.

Weismer G (1984a). Acoustic descriptions of dysarthric speech: perceptual correlates and physiological inferences. Seminars in Speech and Language 5: 293–313.

Weismer G (1984b). Articulatory characteristics of Parkinsonian dysarthria; segmental and phase-level timing, spirantization and glottal-supraglottal co-ordination. In McNeil MR, Rosenbek JC, Aronson AE (eds) The Dysarthrias: Psychology, Acoustics, Perception, Management. San Diego, CA: College Hill, pp.101–30.

Westbrook C, Kaut C (1993). MRI in Practice. Oxford: Blackwell.

Westbury J (1994). X-ray Microbeam Speech Production Database: User's Handbook Version 1.0, Madison, WI: University of Winsconsin.

Wohlert AB, Goffman L (1994). Human perioral muscle activation patterns. Journal of Speech and Hearing Research 37: 1032–40.

Wood S (1997). Electropalatographic Study of Speech Sound Errors in Adults With Acquired Aphasia. PhD, Queen Margaret College, Edinburgh.

Wrench AA, McIntosh AD, Hardcastle WJ (1996). Optopalatograph (OPG): a new apparatus for speech production analysis. Proceedings of ICSLP 96, Philadelphia, PA: Vol. 3, 1589–92.

Zajac DJ, Yates CC (1997). Speech aerodynamics. In Ball MJ, Code C (eds) Instrumental Clinical Phonetics. London: Whurr, pp.87–118.

Ziegler W, Hoole P (1989). A combined acoustic and perceptual analysis of the tense-lax opposition in aphasic vowel production. Aphasiology 3: 449–63.

Ziegler W, Vogel M, Teiwes J, Ahrndt T (1998). Microcomputer-based experimentation assessments and treatment. In Ball MJ, Code C (eds) Instrumental Clinical Phonetics. London: Whurr, pp.262–91.

Index